Etienne Bourdon

Environmental Enrichment for Human Health

A Salutogenic Vision

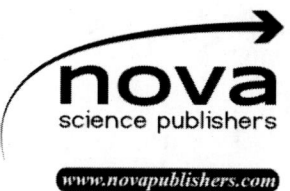

Copyright © 2024 by Nova Science Publishers, Inc.
DOI: https://doi.org/10.52305/YKPU4625

All rights reserved. No part of this book may be reproduced, stored in a retrieval system or transmitted in any form or by any means: electronic, electrostatic, magnetic, tape, mechanical photocopying, recording or otherwise without the written permission of the Publisher.

We have partnered with Copyright Clearance Center to make it easy for you to obtain permissions to reuse content from this publication. Please visit copyright.com and search by Title, ISBN, or ISSN.

For further questions about using the service on copyright.com, please contact:

	Copyright Clearance Center	
Phone: +1-(978) 750-8400	Fax: +1-(978) 750-4470	E-mail: info@copyright.com

NOTICE TO THE READER

The Publisher has taken reasonable care in the preparation of this book but makes no expressed or implied warranty of any kind and assumes no responsibility for any errors or omissions. No liability is assumed for incidental or consequential damages in connection with or arising out of information contained in this book. The Publisher shall not be liable for any special, consequential, or exemplary damages resulting, in whole or in part, from the readers' use of, or reliance upon, this material. Any parts of this book based on government reports are so indicated and copyright is claimed for those parts to the extent applicable to compilations of such works.

Independent verification should be sought for any data, advice or recommendations contained in this book. In addition, no responsibility is assumed by the Publisher for any injury and/or damage to persons or property arising from any methods, products, instructions, ideas or otherwise contained in this publication.

This publication is designed to provide accurate and authoritative information with regards to the subject matter covered herein. It is sold with the clear understanding that the Publisher is not engaged in rendering legal or any other professional services. If legal or any other expert assistance is required, the services of a competent person should be sought. FROM A DECLARATION OF PARTICIPANTS JOINTLY ADOPTED BY A COMMITTEE OF THE AMERICAN BAR ASSOCIATION AND A COMMITTEE OF PUBLISHERS.

Library of Congress Cataloging-in-Publication Data

ISBN: 979-8-89113-623-6 (softcover)
ISBN: 979-8-89113-703-5 (e-book)

Published by Nova Science Publishers, Inc. † New York

Contents

Foreword vii
　　　　　　　Joël Belmin

Acknowledgments xi

General Introduction xiii

Chapter 1　**The Challenges of an Ageing Population** 1
　　　　　　1. The Health of Residents in Institutions 1
　　　　　　2. Alzheimer's Disease and Its Impact on
　　　　　　Institutional Life 3
　　　　　　3. Responses of Geriatric Institutions to the
　　　　　　Challenges of Dementia 4

Chapter 2　**The Influence of the Physical Environment on**
　　　　　　Human Health 7
　　　　　　1. Brief History 7
　　　　　　2. Environmental Concerns of Society 7
　　　　　　3. Promoting a Healthy Environment 8
　　　　　　4. The Challenges and Opportunities for Improving
　　　　　　the Environment in Nursing Homes 10

Chapter 3　**The Physical Environment in**
　　　　　　Geriatric Institutions 13
　　　　　　1. Historical Data and Evolution of Ideas 13
　　　　　　　　1.1. Strong Societal Expectations 13
　　　　　　　　1.2. History of the Physical Environment
　　　　　　　　of Nursing Homes 14
　　　　　　　　1.3. The Green House Project 18
　　　　　　　　1.4. Dementia-Friendly Environment 19
　　　　　　　　1.5. The Enabling Environment 20
　　　　　　　　1.6. Alzheimer Villages 20

Contents

      2. Conceptual Background 22
           2.1. Buber's vision... 22
           2.2. Rogers' Model 23
           2.3. Theories from Lewin and Lawton 24
           2.4. Ulrich and Evidence-Based Design.................. 25
      3. State of Knowledge on the Role of a Nursing
      Home's Physical Environment 27
           3.1. Dining Room Environment 30
           3.2. Garden & Outdoor Facilities 31
           3.3. Sensory Environment... 32
           3.4. Small- vs Large-Scale Nursing Homes............. 35
           3.5. Other Design Features of
           Nursing Homes... 36

Chapter 4   **The Enriched Environment Concept**..............................41
      1. The Development of Enriched Environment.................41
      2. Enriched Environments Used in Experimental
      Work on the Murine Model 45
      3. Enriched Environment Studies on Humans..................47
           3.1. A Few Studies on Autism 47
           3.2. The Leipzig Study 50
      4. The Enriched Environment Research:
      A Wealth of Knowledge 51

Chapter 5   **Transposition of Environmental Enrichment
                to Humans** 59
      1. The Garden Experiences..60
           1.1. Hanging Gardens of Babylon 60
           1.2. Persian Gardens.. 61
           1.3. Gardens of Chinese Scholars 63
           1.4. The Japanese Gardens on
           Kyushu Island.. 64
           1.5. Mediaeval Gardens 65
           1.6. Andalusian Gardens 66
           1.7. English Gardens 67
      2. Sanatoria..67
      3. The Concept of "Therapeutic Garden" or
      "Healing Garden" 70
      4. The Enriched Garden Concept.......................................72
           4.1. Designation 74
           4.2. Understanding 75

        4.3. *The Attributes of the Enriched Garden*............ 77
        4.4. *Extensions of the Enriched Garden*................ 78
   5. Enriched Gardens - Operational Dimensions 79
        5.1. *Enriched Gardens:*
        A Permanent Invitation... 79
        5.2. *Spatial Appropriation and Health* 82
        5.3. *Closeness and Easy Access*............................... 87
        5.4. *Attractiveness* 89
   6. The Enrichment of the Enriched Garden 91
        6.1. *Serenity Space* 92
        6.2. *Garden Easel*.. 93
        6.3. *Sensory Stimulation*
        Amplification Pyramid.. 94
        6.4. *Garden Sundial*.. 96
        6.5. *Floor Painting* 96
        6.6. *Gardening Corner* 98
        6.7. *Musical Instruments* 99

Chapter 6   **Philosophical Background and Currents of Thought** 101
1. Major Philosophical Theories Supporting the Enriched Environment..101
2. Scientific Relativism..104
3. Impoverished Environments...105

Chapter 7   **Enriched Environments: Potential Benefits for Human Health**...109
1. The First Transposition Study of Enriched Environment in Geriatric Institution.................................109
        1.1. *Settings* 109
        1.2. *Intervention* 110
        1.3. *Training the Health Professionals*.................. 112
        1.4. *Measures* 112
        1.5. *Participants* 114
        1.6. *Results* 115
        1.7. *Discussion* 117
        1.8. *Limitations*... 119
2. Conclusions and Implications for Future Development 120

Chapter 8	**Enriched Environments: Spatial Appropriation and Health Benefits** 123	
	1. Introduction 123	
	2. Being at Home - The Notion of Spatial Appropriation 125	
	3. A Qualitative Observational Study of Appropriation with Nursing Home Alzheimer's Residents 127	
	3.1. Selection Criteria 127	
	3.2. Participants 128	
	3.3. Data Collection 129	
	3.4. Data Analysis 129	
	3.5. Results 130	
	3.6. Discussion 135	
	3.7. Limitations and Biases 136	
	Conclusion 136	
Chapter 9	**Enriched Environments: Extension and Perspectives** 139	
	1. Enriched Environments and Older Adults: Perspectives 140	
	2. Enriched Environments and Autism Spectrum Disorder 145	
	3. Further Extensions for Enriched Environments 146	
	4. The Enriched Environment at Home 148	
	5. Enriched Environments in City Centres 149	
	6. The Enriched Environment in a Professional Environment 150	
	Conclusion 151	
References	 153	
Index	 167	

Foreword

Joël Belmin, Professor, MD, PhD
Geriatrician, Faculty Professor at Sorbonne University,
Member of the French Academy of Medicine

The different cultures of mankind have taught us that certain environments provide people with a sense of physical well-being and peace of mind. Gardens, fountains, sounds, smells and architectural features of these environments are just a few examples that obviously contribute to these settings. It's exciting to see that today these themes are being revisited by scientific research. A number of studies have even shown that wellbeing and psychological status of individuals can be positively influenced by favourable environments. In addition, researchers have observed significant associations between features of the physical environment and health outcomes suggesting that a favourable environment might influence not only wellbeing but also the course of diseases and human health. The concept of a healing environment has emerged and is the subject of investigation and research. Conversely, numerous studies have also shown that unfavourable environments, particularly toxic or polluted ones and heat waves, have harmful effects on human health.

Ideas about the healing effects of favourable environments can potentially have a considerable impact on human health. The burden of chronic disease is enormous and increasing despite advances in medical research and access to care, mainly due to the global increase in the number of elderly people. The consequences are not just for individuals, but also for public health, including healthcare organizations, and the economic burden. Conventional therapeutic approaches such as drug treatments, surgery, rehabilitation or psychology have improved the prognosis of many chronic diseases and, on average, these patients are living longer with these diseases. In this context, other new approaches are welcome to improve the course of these chronic diseases and patients' quality of life, and dealing with physical environment could be a promising avenue.

The statistically significant associations between the characteristics of the physical environment and favourable health effects that have been noted in observational studies are not proof of a cause-and-effect relationship. Researchers have all learned that numerous biases can influence the results of their studies, and that these biases may be known or unknown! Evidence of the positive effects of the environment on health can only come from intervention studies. The gold standard for evaluating the effects of a therapy is the double-blind randomized controlled trial, a sophisticated methodology designed to evaluate the effects of a drug compared with a placebo. The implementation of this type of study in humans is very complex for studying the effects of a non-drug treatment, and the same is true for assessing the effects of environments. The methodological challenges involved in designing such studies are considerable. It is very difficult to place individuals in specific, carefully controlled environments for a sufficient period of time, and to assess their effects with complete objectivity, ideally by an assessor who is unaware of the type of environment to which the participants are exposed. Finally, physical environments are always complex, and it would be interesting to know which components of the environment have favourable effects, and which do not. The concept of the enriched environment emerged from this research and is based on the notion that the natural environment can be intentionally modified to have positive effects on the health of the individuals exposed to it. Studies on environmental enrichment are guiding us towards practical, concrete actions that can be implemented in the field, thereby encouraging health promotion based on these concepts.

Of course, the conclusions drawn from these approaches may also be of great interest in preventing these diseases and contributing to healthy ageing.

The book presented by Etienne Bourdon tackles these issues through evidence-based approaches to the effects of the physical environment on health. This book is aimed at caregivers, offering them a new dimension in their practice by associating the major role of the environment. It is addressed to managers of healthcare facilities, underlining the urgent need to question the negative influence of the environment when it can be perceived as an impoverished environment. It provides architects with an essential guideline to integrate into their work on the design or renovation of care facilities. It is addressed to urban planners, sociologists, environmentalists, business leaders and politicians, inviting them to reconsider the physical environment in its influence on human health - whether in geriatric institutions, hospitals, urban spaces, communities, industrial sites or corporate headquarters. Finally, it is aimed at students and all citizens wishing to establish a relationship with their living environment that will have a lasting influence on their health and well-being.

This book marks a major paradigm shift, with the environment on the one hand and health on the other. Rather than considering the environment as an external parameter to be managed, in order to limit its potentially negative influences, which can be assimilated either to natural disasters or to human pollution and nuisance, it draws up a picture of its intimate relationship with our brain's neurotransmitters, and the latter's capacity to compensate for its fragilities. Similarly, the traditionally pathogenic vision is complemented here by a salutogenic approach, inviting society to build a harmonious relationship with the environment, based on prevention and health promotion.

Acknowledgments

Writing this book was a real joy, made up of intense emotions and aspirations to translate them into the production of useful knowledge. To achieve this, I had to learn and question what I thought I knew, and I can't go any further without thanking all those who contributed with relevance, perseverance and kindness.

To Professor Joël Belmin, who combines so many human qualities with a great scientific mind that it's impossible to distinguish one from the other. The enthusiasm and support he has shown me along the way have encouraged me to go even further. His rigor and expertise provided me with such a wealth of support that it made every situation in which I had to question myself a pleasure. Over the years, he has opened my mind like a window, adding a wonderful smile to the horizon,

To John Zeisel, who gave me the benefit not only of his expertise, but also of a rich intellectual and scientific dynamic. His suggestions and highly relevant opinions have given this work essential insights,

To Sylvie Pariel, Alain Koskas, Christophe Bouché, Bruno Oquendo, Christel Oasi, Imani Ramazzani, Julien Meimon, Rachel Pomareis, Sylvain Lavelle and all my colleagues at Charles Foix Hospital and the Sorbonne Paris Nord University laboratory, whose expertise and regular contributions have made a decisive contribution to this research.

And of course, to all the others who are dear to me, whether family or friends, and to whom I owe so much!

General Introduction

The environment and human health have a fragile relationship. Sometimes magnified for the sublime beauty of nature, sometimes feared for the violence of the elements or the harm it can produce, the environment forms the basis of human daily life with this strange paradox between fascination and fear. However, people have always believed that the environment and health are closely linked. As early as the 4th century BC, Hippocrates wrote in his Treaty "On Airs, Waters, and Places" that in order to develop medicine, it is necessary to understand *"due regard to the seasons of the year, and the diseases which they produce, and to the states of the wind peculiar to each country and the qualities of its waters...the localities of towns, and of the surrounding country, whether they are low or high, hot or cold, wet or dry...and of the diet and regiment of the inhabitants."*

The Hippocratic paradox was built on a fatalistic doctrine, accepting the role of the environment while admitting that it could not be changed. A doctrine that imposed submission to the rules of nature without requiring humans to respect it.

Over the centuries, science and medicine have developed alongside human activities, with recommendations on "the hygiene needed in the urban environment, or the impact of deforestation on the healthiness of marshes." The challenges of environmental adaptation were formulated in terms of health concerns - air and water quality in particular in cities, but also waste management, which was a source of multiple epidemics. This concern took on greater reality with the bacteriological work of Koch and Pasteur at the end of the 19th century. This quest for an environmental policy driven by a vision of public health saw the parallel development of environmentalist movements that focused more on enhancing the value of nature, particularly in the urban environment. This was the case in Great Britain with the Green Belt Act initiative in 1938.

Even before a notion of ecology was born, social representations and public health policies associated the environment with the perception of healthy environments. This healthiness was linked not only to the quality of water, air and soil, but also to the way humans managed natural spaces.

In the 19th century, with the development of industrial activities, health policies showed that people were becoming aware of the need to limit deforestation in order to preserve air quality. European countries encouraged intensive reforestation programmes with this aim in mind. These one-off efforts did not stop the continuous assault on the environment by human activities. Whether it was automobile exhaust fumes, pesticides in agriculture, industrial pollution of air and rivers, or the unhealthy housing that was multiplying in the cities, nations paid little attention to the health impacts of these activities. The liberalisation of the economy directly affected the health of workers in various industrial sectors. It was not until the end of the 19th century that the first treatises on industrial hygiene were published, and even then, the purpose of these documents was more to assess the effect of the industrial environment on the health of employees than to promote health policies [1]. The number of subjects reflecting the awareness of the effect of the environment on human health increased during the 20th century. Occupational medicine, which emerged in Europe before the Second World War, sought to prevent the hiring of workers who were likely to develop compensable occupational diseases.

However, whatever the field, the view of the environment in relation to health was associated with a pathogenic vision[2].

This pathogenic view consists of identifying chronic diseases according to their prevalence. This prevalence directs efforts to improve the environment as soon as the origin of a disease is attributed to it. Examples include exposure to asbestos fibres and the risk of developing mesothelioma of the pleura and bronchopulmonary cancers, malaria and the presence of a humid environment favourable to the development of Anopheles mosquitoes, chemical substances, pesticides, air and water pollution, and ultraviolet radiation. The World Health Organization estimates that 13 million people die each year as a result of environmental health hazards, accounting for nearly a quarter of all deaths worldwide [3]. Pathogenesis structures public health policies and seeks to identify the genes, lifestyles, risk factors and, in particular, environmental factors associated with the development of disease. It strives to provide a measured response according to the risks and prevalence of the identified diseases, the means of prevention and the available therapies.

In contrast, salutogenesis, first described by Antonovsky [4] , focuses on factors that promote health and well-being. Salutogenesis focuses on the origins of human health and produces a comprehensive approach to health promotion centred on a positive perception of health, in its relation to the socio-ecological resources, life course and environment that it employs. The term salutogenesis applies to all individual and collective aspects that contribute to the vitality, mental health and well-being of individuals, with a permanent quest for coherence.

This book presents a response that is compatible with this salutogenic vision as a result of a transposition of the research work carried out on enriched environments. Environmental enrichment is a concept described by the neuropsychologist Donald Hebb [5] in 1951 and has been explored almost exclusively on the animal model over the subsequent decades. The research work on enriched environments has highlighted the positive role and effect of enriched environments on brain plasticity.

Hebb's pioneering work highlighted this phenomenon, revealing in particular a greater ability of mice exposed to an enriched environment to 'problem solve' - a process he explained by writing *"when an axon of Cell A is near enough to excite a Cell B and repeatedly or persistently takes share in firing it, some growth process or metabolic change takes place in one or both cells such that A's efficiency, as one of the cells firing B, is increased."* Hebb's starting point was to try to distinguish the physiological and/or psychological origins of behaviour. He focused on analysing the functioning of the brain to explain variations in human behaviour to complement the analysis produced by a psychological approach. The conclusions confirmed by technological progress, particularly in brain imaging, established in particular that the scale of the cerebral cortex changed under the influence of the environment. These observations were extended over the following decades and have been built upon up to the present day by thousands of publications produced by neurobiology laboratories throughout the world. This research investigated not only the effects of the environment on many chronic diseases, but also the way enriched environment impacts the structure and physiology of the brain. All of this work has been central to the inspiration that has guided our studies.

The World Health Organization stated in its World Report on Ageing and Health [6] that "a suitable physical environment can make a difference and is particularly important for older people." However, as we will see in the chapter on the physical environment in geriatric institutions, the many studies that have been carried out have not produced clear recommendations for promoting and preserving the health and quality of life of older people. With regard to general architecture, collective spaces (lounges, restaurants, activity rooms), individual rooms or outdoor spaces, and sensoriality, the studies published throughout the world in recent decades do not converge towards precise guidelines. Although these publications emphasise the significant role of the environment, they fail, mainly for methodological reasons, to set out any guidelines for the health and well-being of nursing home residents.

Studies on enriched environments have produced significant positive responses in many areas of interest in geriatrics - whether it be Alzheimer's disease, Parkinson's disease, depression, disruptive behavioural disorders, cognitive disorders, social bonding, loss of autonomy or chronic pain. Observations made on laboratory mice exposed to an enriched environment compared to a normal or impoverished environment led to the conclusion that the environment has a restorative, compensatory role on age-related pathologies and disorders. Despite the wealth of knowledge acquired over the latter part of the 20th century, clinicians did not seem to have taken hold of the subject, so that no-one took the step of transposing this work from the mouse model to older humans. This work presents the results of the first approach to transposing research on enriched environments to the living environment of older adults in geriatric institutions. The choice of the field of experimentation was oriented towards nursing home gardens in order to free itself from the normative constraints of interior architecture. Because of their cultural heritage and social construction, gardens have a positive image. A garden is capable of accommodating residents in a differentiated space, freeing them from architectural requirements without having to resort to excessive financial resources to adapt it to the specifications of the enriched environment. This is how the concept of the "enriched garden" was formulated - a space for experimentation and the transposition of a concept that had previously been designed for rats and mice. The ethics of respect for people, and in particular the older adults, adopted at the outset of this research programme required maximum distance from the work carried out on the mouse model. This is why it is more appropriate to speak of inspiration than transposition.

The observations made at the end of this initial work have generated considerable enthusiasm among the investigating teams. In studies of institutionalised residents with advanced Alzheimer's disease, it is rare to obtain results that show significant improvement in cognitive abilities or functional autonomy. The methodological rigour adopted in this work, and the wealth of knowledge accumulated by previous studies on the animal model, give rise to great hopes for the interest of continuing the transposition exercise to the various dimensions associated with ageing.

The final chapter of this work outlines, within the framework of a salutogenic vision, the prospects for extending the concept of enriched environment to various areas of human convergence. Thus, we will identify pilot studies and possibilities for enriching the urban space where older adults, people with or without disabilities, children and their parents, and working people meet in order to offer them an environment that promotes and preserves their health. Similarly, enriching the home can help preserve the independence of the older adults and delay the time when they have to leave home for a nursing home. Finally, the workplace, where the multiplicity of occupational illnesses observed through musculoskeletal disorders and psychosocial risks (stress, anxiety, burn-out, depression) can benefit from an enrichment likely to promote a health prevention policy.

Chapter 1

The Challenges of an Ageing Population

The ageing of the world's population observed during the 20th century and the last two decades is an unprecedented phenomenon in human history. The increase in the number of older adults is closely associated with the increase in life expectancy and the growth of the entire population. The decline in the birth rate also contributes to the ageing of the population. These developments have profoundly changed societies, and in particular their health systems. These developments have led to an increase in the number of specialised accommodation facilities, such as long-term care facilities, care homes or nursing homes (NH) in English-speaking countries and establishments for dependent older adults (EHPAD or nursing homes) in France. In 2018, these facilities represented a capacity of more than 6.5 million beds in the countries of the Organization for Economic Co-operation and Development (OECD) [7], with projections indicating a doubling of needs by 2050 (Table 1):

Table 1. Key figures on ageing in OECD countries in 2022 and their projection to 2050

Indicators	2022 (Millions of persons)	2050 (Millions of persons)
+ 65 years	747	1,548
+ 80 years	150	427
Number of Persons with Alzheimer disease	55	139
Number of NH residents	6.5	13

1. The Health of Residents in Institutions

The health of very old people in institutions is characterised by a high prevalence of disability, dependency and multiple chronic diseases, including neurocognitive diseases. Geriatrics, or the medicine of the older adults, studies health in old age; in particular, it aims to identify in complex health states the interactions between natural physiological ageing, chronic or acute diseases and their consequences, and lifestyle, including exposure to deleterious environments.

Table 2. Prevalence of some disorders and diseases of residents in geriatric institutions, according to different sources

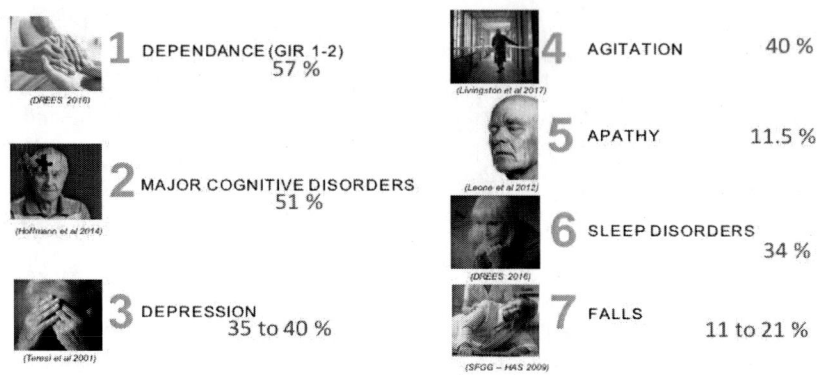

Residents in geriatric institutions present certain clinical situations, called geriatric syndromes, consisting of chronic vulnerability factors (also called predisposing factors) and acute factors that lead to decompensation[1] (also called precipitating factors) [8]. Geriatric syndromes include dependency, malnutrition, gait and balance disorders, depression, mental confusion and chronic neurocognitive disorders, and incontinence. Almost all residents have one or more geriatric syndromes. The origin of geriatric syndromes is multifactorial and can result from the effects of ageing and acute or chronic diseases. Certain diseases associated with old age are common, in particular cataracts, age-related macular degeneration, hearing loss, osteoarthritis, diabetes, cardiovascular disease, chronic obstructive pulmonary disease, Alzheimer's disease and certain cancers. The carer's response is complicated by the multiplicity of disorders observed, the difficulty of establishing a complete history when faced with vulnerable people or people with cognitive losses presenting a complex history. The therapeutic response is limited by the risk of adverse effects associated with poly-medication (iatrogenic effects). The carer must therefore make trade-offs, favouring certain therapeutic approaches according to the expected benefits of each prescription in order to

---

[1] Signs and symptoms of acute deterioration may include, but are not limited to, changes in respiratory rate, oxygen saturation, heart rate or rhythm, blood pressure, mental state, skin perfusion, urine output, or temperature.

improve the patient's daily life. The prevalence of frequent disorders and diseases among residents of geriatric institutions is summarised in Table 2.

These elements underline the complexity of the health problems of this population and their considerable vulnerability.

2. Alzheimer's Disease and Its Impact on Institutional Life

Alzheimer's disease and major neurocognitive disorders are very common among residents of geriatric institutions. Alzheimer's disease was described by the psychiatrist Alois Alzheimer in 1906 based on the observation of a young patient who slowly developed progressive cognitive changes [9]. More than a century later, Alzheimer's disease is one of the most common age-related chronic diseases. For a long time, chronic diseases affecting cognition were referred to as forms of dementia, but today they are referred to as major neurocognitive disorders, since this terminology is more neutral and has less negative connotations than dementia. Alzheimer's disease results from several neuropathological processes involving the formation of amyloid plaques in the extracellular space of the brain. In addition, abnormal changes in tau proteins occur in neurons, altering their role in stabilizing microtubules and leading to the accumulation of neurofibrillary clusters. Other processes such as inflammation of glial cells are involved, and ultimately neuronal death and brain atrophy occur affecting the entire cortex and hippocampus. These neuropathological processes develop slowly and progressively over several decades without causing any symptoms (asymptomatic phase). As these processes develop, symptoms and clinical signs will appear, referred to as the symptomatic phase - (The symptomatic phase includes the mild neurocognitive disorder related to Alzheimer's disease in the first instance, and subsequently the major neurocognitive disorder related to Alzheimer's disease). The major neurocognitive syndrome is defined by the existence of dysfunctions of several cognitive functions concerning memory and at least one other cognitive impairment (executive function, language, praxis, gnosis, attention), and a decline in autonomy with an impact on social relationships [10]. The circumstances in which the disease is discovered, and which lead the patient to consult a doctor are very diverse. The symptoms concerning memory relate to the loss of recent events and are sometimes minimised by the patients and emphasised by their relatives. Many other symptoms are possible, such as language and attention problems, but also non-cognitive symptoms such as repeated falls, weight loss or dependence defined by the need for human assistance for certain activities of daily living. Finally, the disease can be responsible for behavioural changes with so-called negative (apathy) or positive (aggression, agitation, screaming, running away, aberrant motor behaviour, delusions) behavioural disorders often associated with a depressive state [11]. Disruptive behavioural disorders are a major turning point in the evolution of this disease because they make life at home and the involvement of family carers very difficult. Behavioural issues are one of the main reasons for being admitted into a geriatric institution. Numerous publications report the repercussions of these behavioural disorders on family carers, generating fatigue, sleep disorders and anxiety [12]. These behavioural problems represent a major disruption to life in an institution, for residents, carers and relatives during their visits.

3. Responses of Geriatric Institutions to the Challenges of Dementia

Many changes have been made to adapt geriatric institutions to residents suffering from Alzheimer's disease, but they have their limits. Units dedicated to Alzheimer's disease or related disorders, welcome residents in the advanced or severe stages of the disease when they present disruptive behavioural problems. These specialised living units, called Alzheimer's Units, Protected Living Units or Special Care Units, are in fact a sector within a larger institution and are generally designed as small units compared to the rest of the geriatric institution. Grouping together a dozen or so residents, they have undergone significant development and are subject to specific regulations focusing on safety issues - particularly in the management of the movement of people (doors with access codes or secure locks). The staff assigned to them are supposed to have specific training in dealing with behavioural disorders. Kok, Berg and Scherder [13] carried out a systematic review of 32 published studies on special care units and found no significant benefits to the health or quality of life of residents. Gruneir, Lapane and Miller [14] conducted a survey in 2008 of 1519 nursing homes in the USA. Comparing facilities with and without special care units, they found no significant difference in the health status of residents and quality of care. These examples underline the importance of efforts to address the challenges of people with Alzheimer's disease, and the low level of results achieved. A working group led by the Gérontopole de Toulouse [15] drew up an inventory of these special

Alzheimer's units in France and pointed out that "despite continued interest in these structures in the United States, there is still no consensus on the characteristics and specific features of such units." This report notes that "staffing ratios seem to vary widely in Special Care Units, most often higher than in traditional units, but not all studies agree. On the other hand, the time that staff spend directly with patients in Special Care Units is not always greater than in traditional units." Finally, it questions the ethical dimension raised by the deprivation of liberty resulting from the control of access in Special Care Units. If these units do not provide a benefit to the health of the resident, they constitute a system of exclusion likely to feed the feeling of confinement and amplify behavioural problems.

Roger [16] described the high level of medicalisation required by a growing share of residents as "not compatible with an environment favourable to quality of life." The overlap between living, care and working areas creates a conflict of uses within the nursing homes. Few care assistants have specialised in gerontological care to become gerontological care assistants. When they do, they often have little time to develop their skills and must limit themselves to performing primary tasks [17]. Added to this is the difficulty these institutions have in recruiting staff, given the unattractive image and salary. Marquier, Vroylandt and Chenal [18] noted this in a 2016 report by the Directorate for Research, Studies, Evaluation and Statistics (DREES), following a survey over 30 nursing homes.

Faced with an increasingly dependent public, carers often find themselves pushed to the limits of their capacities, faced with the challenge of preserving the function of nursing homes as a place to live. The notion of "pressure of the clock" and "work prevented" due to organisational constraints is described, reflecting a feeling of powerlessness on the part of professionals in the face of users' expectations. Often faced with the challenge of increasing budgetary allocations for staff, public health policies are struggling to meet staffing needs, which, according to demographic projections, are likely to be increasing rapidly in the short term [19].

The successive crises that have arisen in France in recent years have highlighted the significant gap between societal expectations and the reality of daily life and care. For example, the numerous articles published in the public press following the confinement of residents to their rooms in 2020 in connection with the Covid-19 pandemic, or the uproar caused by the publication of the book "Les fossoyeurs: révélations sur le système qui maltraite nos aînés"[2][20], implicating nursing homes run by the ORPEA Group. Nursing homes suffer from a negative image in society and are not managing to improve that image at present.

---

[2] "The gravediggers: revelations about the system that mistreats our elderly."

Chapter 2

The Influence of the Physical Environment on Human Health

The term "physical environment" refers to architectural dimensions such as the interior and exterior of a geriatric institution, as well as the furniture and the resulting sensory elements such as natural or artificial light, sounds, textures and scents.

1. Brief History

There has always been a belief that environment and health are closely linked. Today, people take it for granted that their relationship with the environment is essential to their health. This link has been forged under the influence of cultural, political, philosophical and economic considerations, as well as scientific ones, and in particular public health factors. In the 15th and 16th centuries, the manuscripts of Jones in England [21] and the texts of Villermé [22] in France emphasised the need to take care of the urban environment in order to limit public health risks. In contrast to the "Enlightenment," which celebrated the triumph of reason and civilization, the Romantic movement asserted that the contemplation of 'nature' was a source of universal harmony. The opposition in 19th-century England and France between utopians and reformists in the face of the development of industrialisation, as described by Mathis (1), is summed up with the question "*should natural places be preserved for the people or from the people?*" An article by Wilkinson, Smith and Davies, which raises the issue of reducing greenhouse gases as a public health issue, was not published by the Lancet until 2009 [23].

2. Environmental Concerns of Society

It was often when people realised the harmful effects of exposure to a harmful environment that they realised they had to take care of it. The emergence of pandemics linked to water quality, the impact of deforestation on air quality, and the impact of coal fumes in urban areas are all examples of situations that made people aware that they had to build a balanced relationship with the environment.

This environmental concern has manifested itself in the organisation of global conferences by the United Nations. The first United Nations Conference on the Human Environment [24], held in Stockholm in 1972, resulted in the following declaration: *".../... We have reached a point in history where we must shape our actions throughout the world with greater caution about their environmental consequences. Through ignorance or indifference, we can cause massive and irreversible damage to the earth's environment on which our lives and well-being depend. Conversely, with greater knowledge and wiser action, we can achieve for ourselves and our posterity a better life in an environment more in keeping with human needs and hopes."* The essence of this joint declaration is the need to limit environmental pollution from human activities. The Stockholm conference highlighted the impact of industrialised countries on developing countries. The environmental concern of people, politicians and scientific communities has grown over the decades, gradually positioning the issue as a matter of survival for humanity and the planet. Environmental health issues have been approached essentially from the perspective of reducing harm.

3. Promoting a Healthy Environment

Building a relationship with the environment in order to improve human health is an idea developed by Antonovsky in 1979 through his theory entitled Salutogenesis. Public health issues are usually considered with the aim of preventing the development of pathologies (pathogenesis). In contrast to this "pathogenic" view, Antonovsky proposes to highlight the factors that will promote people's health. Salutogenesis is based on the search for the origins of health. It is an approach that induces a notion of coherence in the quest for well-being and physical and mental health: "*it suggests that all salutogenic processes are channelled through a measurable global life orientation*"[25]. The challenge posed by Salutogenesis, in this world where so many "*potentially pathogenic agents*" surround us, is to focus on the essentials, namely "*what makes us alive and provides us with well-being.*" According to Antonovsky, to focus on pathologies is to handicap humanity by posing both the scientific problem of solving them and the moral problem of reducing pain and suffering. The pathogenic logic is part of a comfortable logic based on one disease = one therapy. The pathogenic model postulates the pathological state, in contrast to the salutogenic model which is built around the healthy individual. The theory of Salutogenesis, which was initiated more than 40 years ago, is updated every year by a group of researchers in biomedicine, public health and social sciences, namely the Global Working Group on Salutogenesis, which works to defend the quest for well-being and the scientific approach that accompanies it. Thus Becker, Glascoff and Felts [26], 30 years after the development of the concept of Salutogenesis, observe that the reduction of negative health states associated with "Pathogenesis" does not necessarily increase positive states. They propose combining the two approaches - Pathogenesis and Salutogenesis - to create a physical environment that both reduces the occurrence of major chronic diseases and supports and nurtures a strategy of health and well-being.

The concept of therapy in relation to the use of a health-promoting environment was described in the work of Kaplan and Kaplan. In their book "*The experience of nature: A psychological perspective,*" they developed "*the Attention restoration theory*"[27]. The authors describe this essentially psychological capacity for restoration as bringing new understanding to the role of the environment on health. When an environment has certain characteristics such as fascination, unusualness, invitation to reverie, and compatibility, it is likely to reduce stress and mental fatigue. It is in the early 80's as well that environmental psychology was formalised, dealing with ecological and architectural issues as well as social relations between individuals. Environmental psychology is based on the work of the psychologist Lewin [28] who developed the field theory in which behaviour depends on the person and his environment. These founding approaches found an extension in many fields, such as those brought by Lawton who was interested in the role of the environment on the health of the older adults, underlining its importance in the preservation of autonomy.

The juxtaposition of these approaches, those conducted by the United Nations conferences for the environment and those conducted by the scientists mentioned above, suggest two different relationships to the environment. One invites us to take care of it in order to limit the negative effects on health (Pathogenesis), the other encourages us to enhance it in order to promote quality of life (Salutogenesis). What environmental approach should be adopted in order to limit the pollution that is harmful to health on the one hand, while at the same time developing a living environment that is likely to cure disorders and restore certain faculties?

4. The Challenges and Opportunities for Improving the Environment in Nursing Homes

The perception of the role played by the physical environment on human health has had many repercussions on the development of geriatric institutions. Consideration has been given to defining the ideal living environment to accompany the critical phases of ageing [29]. Should the concept of nursing homes be abandoned? Should we design an architecture for these establishments that is further away from hospital logic while still being able to provide the care and assistance required when a person presents multiple pathologies and dependencies? How can the environment best support these challenges by contributing to the quality of life and health of the residents? [30-31] These considerations also generate expectations regarding environmental adaptations within special Alzheimer's units where the secure setting, motivated by a desire to prevent risks related to running away and wandering, is emphasised to the detriment of freedom of movement [32].

It is in this context that, for several decades, numerous teams have undertaken major research efforts to describe and optimise the physical environment of these establishments [33]. From this work, there are no widely accepted notions about the types of physical environment that should be promoted in geriatric institutions. Therefore, we conducted a review of the literature to identify environmental factors that can have a positive effect on the health of residents in institutions.

Work consisting of intervening on the environment and enriching it to positively influence health caught our attention. The concept of environmental enrichment [34] provides a source of information that can inspire the search for the ideal living environment for the older adults in institutions.

Sidebar 1. The enriched environment

Environmental enrichment is a result of the pioneering work of Hebb. In 1946, Hebb demonstrated that rats raised as pets had greater problem-solving skills than their caged counterparts. Subsequently, the construction of cages with play elements (wheels, ladders, walkways) showed the impact of the environment on brain activity. The concept of an enriched environment has become established as a device for studying the environment on the brain's perception centres and their effect on health.

Studies conducted on the mouse model have explored the effects of an enriched environment, particularly on mice suffering from cognitive disorders, Alzheimer's disease, and Parkinson's disease.

These scientific experiments using the enriched environment as a research model are an important source of inspiration for the development of the geriatric field.

Among the existing spaces in geriatric institutions, gardens were identified as spaces of well-being because of their proximity to nature.

Gardens were opened and became an important part of nursing homes and were often designated as Alzheimer's gardens, sensory gardens or therapeutic gardens. These gardens were established in the green spaces around the buildings or, when there was not enough green space, they were laid out in patios or on terraces. The heritage of gardens evokes philosophical, sociological, political, cultural and religious representations of the human ideal. Gardens have very often been associated with the practice of traditional medicine, particularly through the cultivation of medicinal plants by monks. Over the centuries, gardens have retained their image as a healthy and virtuous space that accompanies human constructions, so much so that in November 2014, the Minister of the Environment Ségolène Royal [35] declared: *"we are going with the Minister of Health (Marisol Touraine) to make these therapeutic gardens a standard feature in all establishments that treat patients with Alzheimer's disease."* Gardens in institutions have however been limited by low attendance and the weak confirmation of the benefits on the health of the residents.

The work presented in this thesis is part of this quest for a balanced relationship between the environment and health.

Combining concerns about the frailties, disorders and pathologies of older adults living in medico-social institutions, the work carried out in recent decades on the quantifiable links between the environment of a nursing home and the quality of life and health of residents, the knowledge acquired by scientific research on the enriched environment, but also the experiences of therapeutic gardens set up in certain establishments, the benefits of the innovative concept of "enriched gardens" has become apparent.

Can an enriched garden, which forms a specific territory at the frontiers of ageing, health and environmental research, become a place where all the expectations of nursing homes can be monitored or a place where the well-being and quality of life of the resident can be revealed?

The aim of this research is to define the context, the potential and the perspectives in which the principles of environmental enrichment can be extended to the various dimensions of people's physical living environment.

Sidebar 2. The enriched garden

The enriched garden is an innovative concept resulting from the transposition of the enriched environment into the specific space of the garden. The enriched garden is set up in a geriatric institution. The enrichment of the garden is formed by the arrangement of specific "modules" which constitute the active material of the garden. They have been designed according to precise therapeutic objectives corresponding to the disorders and weaknesses observed among the residents (cognitive, behavioural and mood disorders, loss of independence, etc.). The interactions that the resident spontaneously establishes with these modules participate in sensory stimulation intended to produce beneficial effects on his or her health.

The enriched garden is an experimental device aimed at evaluating the links between the physical environment and the health and well-being of residents.

Chapter 3

The Physical Environment in Geriatric Institutions

1. Historical Data and Evolution of Ideas

1.1. Strong Societal Expectations

The challenges of ageing populations have repercussions on life in geriatric institutions. The policy on ageing in France since the Laroque report in 1962 [36] and reaffirmed by the law on the adaptation of society to ageing in 2015, is centred on home care. Although regularly questioned in public debates, nursing homes remain the solution of last resort offered to older adults losing their autonomy. Providing care for these residents constitutes a major challenge today and for decades to come. The growing number of older adults, the tendency to postpone dependency and delay entry into an institution, and the medical skills required to care for them, create an overlap in nursing homes between a place of living and a place of care. What is needed is a familiar and warm environment, capable of promoting free choice and maintaining the functional and decision-making autonomy of individuals. It is a question of thinking about adaptation to disabilities in an integrated way, in a logic of universal design, which does not stigmatise people in the difficulties they encounter. The reference model should be that of the home and not the hospital. In 2021, Champvert [37] expressed his point of view as director of the Association of Directors for the Elderly: "The institutional and support service for the older adults has just shown its limits and now appears to be out of breath. It is therefore imperative that this system integrates a genuine culture of the home, going beyond the outdated, health-centred model and allowing the continuation of life at home to be guaranteed, whatever the form of housing. While enhancing the health mission, it is important to preserve the remaining capacities of residents in an approach that involves all aspects of the establishment: architectural project, establishment project, life project. Beyond the aesthetics or the general architecture of the buildings, it is a question of adopting an integrative vision, with adaptations that are likely to allow the residents to preserve, reinforce or even develop their opportunities to act, their degree of control over their tasks and the way in which they carry them out, that is to say their autonomy. Openness to the environment allows everyone, whatever the difficulties encountered, to be a full citizen, to have access to fulfilling social relations and to formulate projects for themselves. Taking into account the local culture and identity allows people to belong to a territory, by seeking harmony and continuity with the urban environment.

This is important in order to encourage appropriation and familiarity of the site for everyone, both residents of the site and of the town. The expected vision of nursing homes is that of an architectural space that goes beyond the mere functional logic of accommodation premises, to seek a quality of use and atmosphere and create a real habitat that is a source of well-being for all (residents and professionals). This domiciliary logic stated by Champvert does not fundamentally call into question the existence of nursing homes but assumes that it integrates the culture of the home while allowing residents to break with social isolation and limiting the costs of care by a logic of proximity. The work of Havreng-Thery [38] on the quality of care in nursing homes has highlighted the importance of the garden in the expectations of residents and families, without any specific distinction being made with regard to the nature and architectural quality of the garden. The main expectations and visions of today's and tomorrow's nursing homes are thus expressed in conferences, publications and renovation projects.

1.2. History of the Physical Environment of Nursing Homes

1.2.1. The Origin of Nursing Homes in France
Geriatric institutions in France and nursing homes throughout the world have developed in line with the increase in life expectancy, the state of health of the older adults, and the evolution of social protection. The developments that preceded nursing homes reflect the way societies view the older adults. In France, the first structures emerged in the Middle Ages with religiously inspired charitable establishments for the indigent. Under Louis XIV, hospices operated within a logic of exclusion aimed more at removing the indigent from the public arena than at caring for them. It was not until the end of the 18th century that these institutions, based on a logic of exclusion, were transformed into hospices dedicated to the reception of the most destitute, but also of the

'old'. These public or religious hospices[3], where "charity" was practised, saw the appearance of infirmaries towards the middle of the 19th century, making their mission evolve from a social purpose to a combined medical and social purpose. A slow but steady growth of these establishments can be observed until the promulgation of the law of 14 July 1905 [39] on "assistance to the older adults, the infirm and the incurable," which impacted any destitute older adults over 70 years old. According to this legislation, 90% of them received a monthly allowance at home. According to Zanetti and Rossigneux-Méheust [40], "the Catholic Church saw the opportunity to express its values (notably charity) in the face of growing anticlericalism and allowed the Little Sisters of the Poor to found several hundred establishments." Similarly, some large companies rejected a vision of working-class paternalism by creating private hospices. On the eve of the First World War, the state's view of ageing changed, considering that it had a duty to protect the older adults. Initiated in the 19th century, growing urbanisation and the rural exodus, linked to industrialisation, took the older adults out of the private sphere, destabilising the traditional family unit. The architecture of the hospices was supported at this time by the hygienist trend developed in the sanatoriums, favouring the suburban system, but also the distance from the city centre [41]. The period of the "Trente Glorieuses" (1945-1975) was accompanied by a real improvement in the lot of the older adults thanks to various mutual aid measures such as the creation of Social Security in 1945 and the National Solidarity Fund in 1956, and the development of pensions for all, which encouraged people to stay at home. The Laroque report (1962) established home care as a pillar of old age policy. It came at a time dominated by poor housing, social isolation and poverty among those left behind by the growth of the economy. It promoted housing renovation actions. The founding law on care homes dates from 30 July 1975. It decided that hospices should be abolished within 15 years and transformed into health units - this is how care homes came into being. As a result, many care homes were created and their number increased from 1500 in 1975 to 7500 in 2021 [42]. This marked the beginning of a legal and technical transformation of these establishments, which gradually lost their religious dimension and were placed under the supervision of public services. In the early 2000s, these care homes became an available market for the private sector. The discrepancy between demand and the number of places available, and the discrepancy between the quality of care and the expectations

---

[3] The meaning of the word hospice has evolved over the centuries from a place of refuge for travellers to the modern institution for palliative care.

of the public are described by Castel [43] in his book "L'Insécurité sociale[4]." He defines this feeling of insecurity on the part of the older adults and their families when faced with the prospect of entering an institution: "If modern societies are built on a foundation of insecurity, it is because the individuals who live in them do not find, either in themselves or in their immediate environment, the capacity to ensure their protection." It was with the law of 2 January 2002 [44] that the status of care homes changed to that of Establishment for the Dependent Older adults or EHPAD. It is therefore towards these EHPADs, which have received so much criticism, that the accommodation for the "destitute elderly" of the 1905 law has evolved. These changes have accompanied an increase in life expectancy, the break-up of the traditional family circle, which has lost its capacity to accompany the older adults, and an increase in dependency and age-related pathologies, which require professional care.

1.2.2. Nursing Homes and the Health of the Older Adults

The French Ministry of Health's [45] national plan for "Ageing well" (2007-2009) set out the priorities for the care of nursing home residents. These priorities are expressed in the form of recommendations, some of which concern the living conditions and environment. It concluded that care of the older adults must emphasise personalised support, the living environment must allow the resident to appropriate the space of his or her home and to meet other residents, social life must preserve relations with family and friends and favour collective life, and finally, healthcare must aim to limit falls, malnutrition, dehydration, bedsores, infections and incontinence [46].

The capacity of geriatric institutions to respond to the missions defined by the various old age policies and health and social coordination plans is difficult to evaluate [47]. These evaluations mainly focus on the quality of care and rarely on the quality of the physical environment. The High Authority for Health asks: "Do geriatric institutions provide prevention and appropriate care for residents' health, contributing to a good quality of life? The Senate report of 23 February 2022 [48] makes this observation in its session entitled "The medicalization of EHPADs - a new model to be built" - following a survey conducted in 2021 among 57 public, private and cooperative institutions. This report notes that the quality of care provided in institutions does not meet the needs of this poly-pathological and heavily dependent population. Tran, Nguyen and Gray [49] published a literature review on the quality of care in

---

[4] Social insecurity.

nursing homes in 2019. They conclude that the quality of care is relatively infrequently evaluated and that when it is done, evaluations are focused on indicators such as the ratio of caregivers to residents or the level of training of health professionals. The authors point out that only one of the 39 studies reviewed assessed the quality of life of residents in relation to the quality of care provided. These different analyses confirm the difficulty of implementing effective strategies to improve the quality of life of residents in geriatric institutions.

The health mission of nursing homes, which was spelled out in France in the 1975 law, has not been convincingly established. A gap has opened up between the level of services offered and the needs of residents due to the changing profile of the population, the inadequacy of staffing levels and training for carers, and the lack of response and therapeutic follow-up mechanisms - given the complexity of the disorders observed among residents and described in the introduction. While there is a convergence of opinion on the need to renovate the nursing homes model, economic, structural and medical difficulties will increase the complexity of implementing these changes. The role of the environment, although regularly mentioned as a positive factor, is rarely taken into account in its capacity to improve the health and quality of life of residents.

1.2.3. The Role of the Physical Environment in Nursing Homes
The World Health Organization's 2002 report on Ageing and Health [6] states in its introduction that "a suitable physical environment can make the difference between independence and dependence for all individuals, but it is particularly important for older people." Although there is no single architectural model for geriatric institutions, the major OECD countries have set certain limits on the regulatory and budgetary framework for these facilities. These limits include the size and relative proportion of single rooms vs communal space. These rules vary from country to country, depending on historical, economic and cultural factors. In addition to the architectural rules, there are concepts related to the dignity, privacy and safety of the resident. Although, as described above, ageing in institutions has remained a solution of last resort compared to home care, it has always reflected the negative image of the hospital environment, as described in particular in Girard's diary (1722-1795): *"It is undeniable, both at the Hôtel-Dieu and at the general hospital, that the patients sleep several in one bed"*[50]. The heritage of EHPADs in France reflects the history of hospital architecture, with its hospices, sanatoria, dispensaries and hospital services. In France, the 1975 law

on the transformation of hospices into medical or non-medical care homes encouraged the development of establishments in the form of functional buildings in the architectural style of the 1970s and 1980s. These are often multi-storey concrete blocks with long corridors leading to the rooms, which are supposed to facilitate the distribution of care and services. The development of real estate projects for new care homes has been driven by a logic of profitability for investors and has led to the choice of land outside urban areas. The distance of these new establishments from city centres contributes to the feeling of isolation and rupture of social links for many residents.

The 2002 law, which created EHPADs in France, initiated a change in which architecture must adapt to the needs of residents and their carers and no longer be based solely on utilitarian and functional logic. New projects and renovations must reconcile the challenges of creating a place to live, care, work and receive people, while being located as much as possible in the heart of the city. In an article reviewing nursing homes in the United States, Hawes and Charles [51] describe a development of the private sector favoured by the transition to Medicare and Medicaid. According to Hawes, this development, centred on optimizing the legal system in order to maximise profits, is taking place at the expense of the quality of life of residents. This has led to debate and research on the quality of the environment offered to residents in relation to the ownership of facilities. Fottler, Smith and James [52] suggest that there is a conflict between the pursuit of profitability and the design of the environment.

1.3. The Green House Project

An initiative by Dr William Thomas in the USA in 2002, stemming from *the Eden Alternative Concept,* provided a new model for the environment of nursing homes with *the National Green House Project* [53]. The idea was to move from a medicalised model to a social model of long-term care, in which large-scale establishments (more than 100 residents) were converted into 4 or 5 smaller-scale buildings, on a more human scale, inspired by a residential logic. The aim was to promote conviviality in households of 10-12 residents, where meals are taken together and access to a patio or garden is supposed to break with the traditional hospital culture. The nurses were given a new title: *Shahbaz* (in the sense of protector) and received additional training to enable them to extend their scope of responsibility to various daily tasks (cooking, shopping, cleaning, etc.). These *Shahbazim* no longer report hierarchically to the director of the establishment but to a guide and a sage who are independent personalities, trained in the Green House Project, and who check whether the practices comply with the specifications. The active communication around *the Green House Project*, supported in particular by Kane's work [54], helped to spread the concept and in particular the need to change the scale of the establishments by making them evolve towards small-scale, family-type structures.

1.4. Dementia-Friendly Environment

Another approach in favour of the environment is called the "dementia-friendly environment." The World Health Organization has defined it as follows: "*Initiatives for people with dementia should aim to change the physical and social environment to make a community more inclusive, accessible and responsive to older people and people with dementia*"[55]. This concept was initiated by the notion of Person-Centred-Care (PCC) inspired by Lawton's model [56] describing the interactions between the pressure exerted by the environment and an individual's abilities. The first study was conducted by Netten [57] in 1989 on 13 nursing homes. These adaptations were guided by the main disorders identified in the patient, including difficulties with spatial orientation, social relationships, behavioural problems and sensory perception. Marquardt and Schmieg [58] presented a study on the role of the Dementia-Friendly Environment in helping cognitively impaired residents to orient themselves in the institution. Indeed, cognitive impairment decreases the ability to find one's way to one's room, and to get to and from a space. The study showed that in facilities with dementia-friendly architecture, residents' orientation performance (as assessed by nurses) was significantly better than in other facilities. By facilitating orientation, the person with dementia experiences more well-being and presents fewer behavioural problems. Fleming and Bennett [31, 59] presented recommendations for adapting the environment to the *Dementia Friendly Environment concept* with Alzheimer's patients in Australia:

1. Reduce risks by preserving circulation and providing spatial cues.
2. Design the space on a human scale.
3. Allow people to see and be seen.

4. Reduce unnecessary stimulation.
5. Optimise useful stimuli.
6. Promote movement and engagement.
7. Create a familiar space and limit decision making during movement in the space.
8. Provide opportunities to be alone or with others.
9. Strengthen social connection.
10. Adapt to the lifestyle.

1.5. The Enabling Environment

The concept of the "enabling environment," initiated as part of an ergonomic optimisation approach in the world of work, was developed in France in 2005, particularly by Falzon [60]. It is part of a constructive vision of the interaction of individuals with their environment. Its main adaptations have been in the world of work in order to facilitate the learning of new skills or to preserve existing skills. It has found applications both for individual and collective learning, particularly in relation to machines and computer tools. This concept has been extended to the field of physical and mental disability and chronic illness [61].

This approach, translated into the expression "*enabling environment*," has been extended to the interior design of geriatric institutions, with a logic quite similar to that developed in the *dementia-friendly environment*, but with an orientation towards maintaining autonomy. This concept of an enabling environment that is focused on preserving functional independence is based on the search for appropriate ergonomics, signage, lighting, sensory stimuli, multifunctional spaces, intuitiveness and also the reduction of psychosocial risks for health professionals [62].

1.6. Alzheimer Villages

More recently, the creation of Alzheimer's villages has attracted particular attention. The first one was created in the Netherlands in 2009 with the Hogeweyk Dementia Village. The aim is to create an environment with a village atmosphere, which goes beyond the institutional framework to offer an inclusive living environment focused on individuals with Alzheimer's disease. These Alzheimer's villages are designed as a fulfilling and inclusive alternative to geriatric institutions. The architects have received training on the main characteristics of people with Alzheimer's disease. Each village is divided into groups of 8 to 12 residents, and is open to the outside world, a place where residents eat when they want to and not at fixed times. They have shops and cafés where they meet local residents who have free access. Here are some examples of the living environment reported from Hogeweyk village [63]: *"The covered passage smells of freshly baked cookies. Funny conversations can be heard, interrupted for a moment when the oven beeps, in the kitchen which has been decorated in the old-fashioned way. A tray of freshly baked biscuits is pulled from the oven. Two women, one in a wheelchair, enter the place, obviously seduced by the smell.../... On the Boulevard, the copper letters on the façade of the Mozart Hall shine in the sunlight. Classical music can be heard. Through the window, a group of men and women can be seen dancing in the room while others in wheelchairs sway to the music..."* Many other Alzheimer's villages have been set up around the world, in Germany, Switzerland, Great Britain, Denmark, Canada and the United States, but also in France with the village of Dax in the Landes region, which opened in 2019. Overall, they are designed as an experiment to assess whether they constitute a beneficial environment for people with advanced Alzheimer's disease. The studies conducted at the Landes Alzheimer's Village focus on the social involvement of the villagers, the stress levels of the professionals, and the relationships maintained by the carers. No publication has yet been produced from the studies conducted in this village, which are led by the Psycho-epidemiology of Ageing and Chronic Diseases Unit of INSERM. Generally speaking, few studies in this area have been published to date. However, it is worth mentioning the work of Peoples, Pedersen and Moestrup [64] whose conclusions can be summarised as follows: *"The results showed that relatives of people with dementia and health professionals were committed to creating and maintaining a meaningful daily life for residents, but also revealed different perceptions of time and space and how this could be understood and better achieved. In addition, people with advanced dementia may not be able to benefit from the activities and opportunities offered by the Alzheimer's village, as this requires resources beyond what may be available."*

The results of the evaluations of these experiences will help determine whether the Alzheimer's Village concept will become a pathway to follow and multiply in the future.

2. Conceptual Background

This research programme is at the crossroads between the environment and the health of the individual, and particularly the older adults. It is based on a holistic vision of care. Much of the work in this area is part of a Person-Centred-Care approach, which is generally associated with a Person-Centred Environment (PCE) approach. Person-centred care [65] is a philosophy of care that focuses on the needs of the individual and is based on knowing the person through an interpersonal relationship. It challenges the traditional medical model of care which tends to focus on processes, schedules and the needs of staff and the organisation [66]. At the origin of these notions, several founding theories must be considered.

2.1. Buber's Vision

Buber [67] described in a holistic vision the relationship that each individual establishes with his environment. Buber supports the notion that the person does not exist without this relationship and this experience of the world around him. He criticised the modern Enlightenment notion of the subject as a separate, substantial and rational entity, as opposed to a world of 'things-in-themselves' and formulated it only in terms of its dependence on relationships with otherness. Buber summarised his perception of the individual in a triangular relationship (Figure 2) based on a continuous dialogue (verbal or non-verbal) that nourishes his knowledge. The relationship that Buber suggests in medical practice is established primarily not on the expertise and knowledge that the carer possesses, but on the nature of the relationship that is created with the patient: "*I become in touch with you.*" Translating Buber's approach into care practice is to heal where possible, to reduce suffering where healing is not possible and to understand meaning beyond the experience of illness. This relationship in a caregiver/patient exchange is based on a bond of symmetry and reciprocity (Figure 1). Levinas will add to this relationship, an essential question according to him concerning the vulnerability of the patient which obligates the carer to an infinite responsibility.

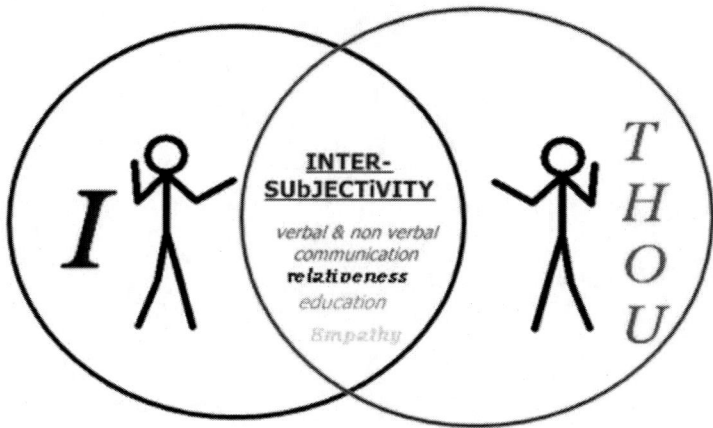

Figure 1. Buber I Thou relationship model.

2.2. Rogers' Model

Rogers' model [68] describes the relationship between the therapist and the patient in the initial context of psychotherapy. It is the foundation of a global approach to person-centred care. Rogers does not place himself in Buber's lineage, although he has dialogued with him on several occasions [69]. His non-directive approach is intended to accompany the patient in his or her evolution and change, which is the motor of his or her inner transformation. Rogers' model was a real innovation in psychotherapy and was a source of inspiration in many fields (Figure 2).

Rogers' holistic and humanistic model goes beyond the specific framework of psychotherapy and inspired the work of Kitwood. This notion of person-centred care was developed by Kitwood in 1988 [31] with Alzheimer's patients to encourage efforts to understand the patient. He advocates a relational construction based on communication in which cognitive disorders are only a transactional factor in addition to the psychosocial dimension, health and personality of the person. Kitwood, inspired by Rogers' model, was convinced of the essential role played by the environment in the construction of the relationship that is established with a person suffering from Alzheimer's disease. Kitwood thus rejected the biomedical model, which consisted of focusing exclusively on the pathophysiological dimension in order to address the human being as a whole [65].

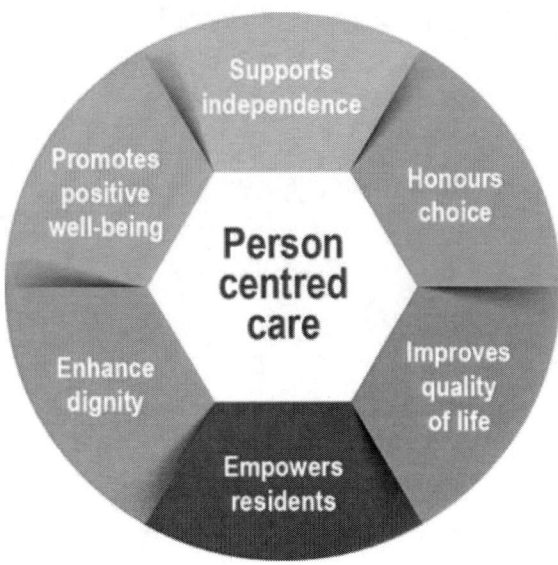

Figure 2. Person-centred care – representation by Mead and Bower (2000) [70].

2.3. Theories from Lewin and Lawton

Lewin (28) on the one hand, and Lawton [56-71] on the other hand, have constructed the relationship between man and the environment in a transactional approach. In this approach, the individual establishes his relationship with reciprocity and a continuous exchange with the environment without being able to really separate one from the other. The analytical effort therefore focuses on understanding the couple that is formed between the two. Lawton analyses this relationship in the context of a reciprocity in which the environment exerts pressure and the individual must mobilise his ability to cope with it by (see Figure 3):

- Cognitive skills,
- His behavioural skills,
- His emotions resulting from his relationship with the environment.

During this relationship, the transaction adapts according to the level of stimulation exerted and the person's capacity to integrate it, producing, depending on the case, a renunciation or an inappropriate behaviour. Lawton based his theory on the equation established by Lewin:

B = f (p, e)

describing behaviour (B) as a combined function of the environment (e) and the person (p). Working on health issues related to ageing, Lawton supplemented this equation with the following formulation:

B = f (P, E (P x E))

taking into account that for a given environment the (P x E) relationship was well defined.

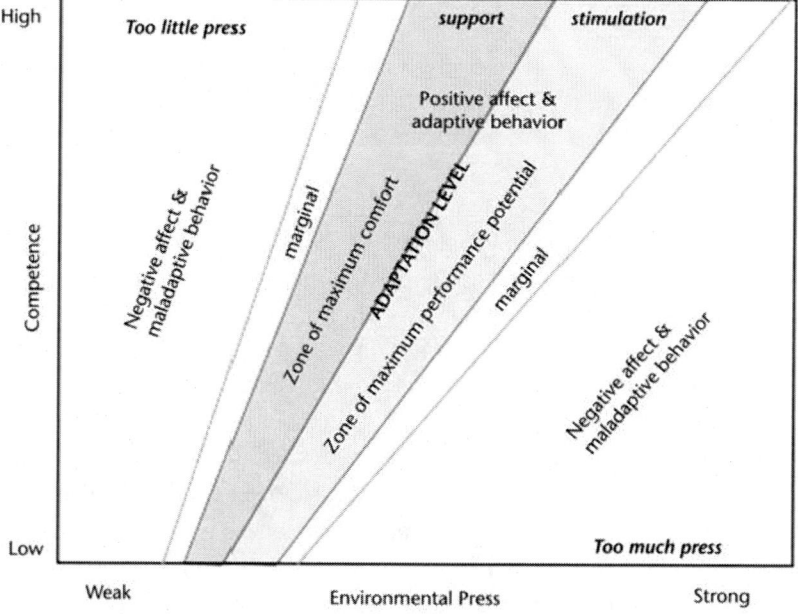

Figure 3. Lawton's ecological model of adaptation and ageing [72].

2.4. Ulrich and Evidence-Based Design

Ulrich [73] has used his work to promote the *Evidence-Based Design* approach. This approach, which has become popular with architects, is based on the main conclusions drawn from the scientific literature, particularly literature reviews, to dictate the practices to be adopted in the design of medico-social establishments [74]. In a literature review, Ulrich, Zimring and Zhu establish *Evidence-Based Design* as a concept capable of providing useful insights into the physical environment in relation to patient safety (including medical errors, infections and falls), patient health (including pain, stress, sleep, length of stay, depression, spatial orientation etc.) and the quality of work life of carers (such as stress, efficiency, musculoskeletal disorders and psychosocial risks) [75]. However, Ulrich has highlighted the relative significance of the conclusions drawn from *Evidence-Based Design*, due to the methodological weakness of the available work, in particular the small number of randomised controlled trials. Evidence-Based Design remains, however, a reference for the implementation of Antonovsky's perspective of Salutogenesis, through its efforts to build an environment conducive to the physical, mental and social well-being of the patient.

This approach was taken up by Grahn and Bengtsson [76], two Swedes who transferred research on the rehabilitative benefits provided by public gardens to the design of gardens in geriatric institutions. They combined *Evidence-Based Design* with environmental quality assessment tools to form a triangulation model to highlight the health benefits for patients. The work of Grahn distinguished between a variety of levels of the patient's relationship with the environment, depending on the more or less passive mode of interaction with the environment. Invoking the work of Kaplan and Kaplan, they associated the benefits of *Attention Restoration Theory* with a passive relationship based on the fascination of the environment. According to them, the healing garden participates in a salutogenic strategy through this passive exercise of contemplation. To ensure the success of salutogenic design, Golembiewski and Zeisel [77] propose considering the resident as a person with abilities and resources, rather than as a patient to be cared for. Grahn [78] have represented their understanding of these relationships that the patient/resident establishes with the institutional environment in a triangle (Figure 4).

The theory of Grahn is based on a combination of a pathogenic strategy, aimed at eliminating risk factors, with a salutogenic strategy based on a permanent invitation to the older adults' residents to enjoy the garden, by increasing the demand for their attention. According to Grahn, this involvement of residents with their environment is a factor in improving their well-being.

The Physical Environment in Geriatric Institutions

Following Grahn, Stigsdotter [79] described that a more active relationship with the environment, based mainly on gardening, contributed more to spatial appropriation[5] and well-being.

These different theoretical frameworks form models for understanding this relationship that humans establish with their environment and the role of the stimuli exerted by the latter.

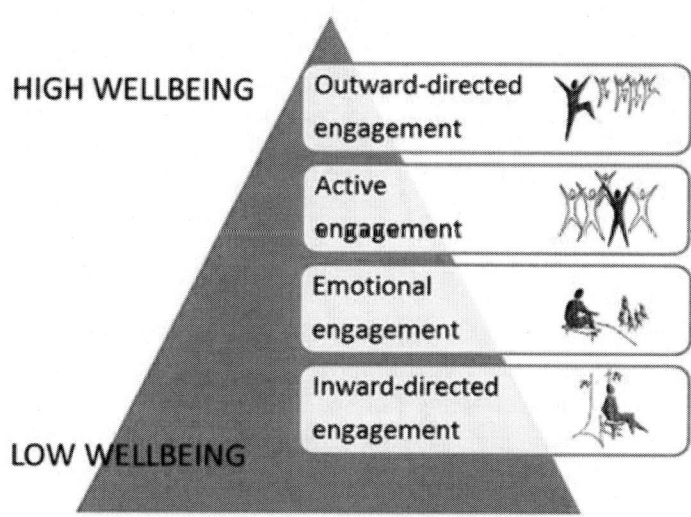

Figure 4. The Grahn triangle of relationships between environment and well-being as a function of resident involvement.

3. State of Knowledge on the Role of a Nursing Home's Physical Environment

These geriatric settings face a major challenge: how to offer care services that respond to the increasing frailty of their residents while at the same time providing a pleasant and adapted living environment in which residents feel well and can invest in new projects. In this respect, numerous publications regularly emphasise that the physical environment is an important factor in determining quality of life (QoL), well-being and health [64].

The role of the physical environment on health has been extensively explored in scientific research, particularly in animal studies. In his pioneering

---

[5] Spatial appropriation describes the many ways in which a visitor considers a space as its own.

intervention studies, neuropsychologist Hebb found that environmental enrichment improved cognitive abilities in mice. Later on, this intervention was found to increase the volume of the cerebral cortex and to produce neurobiological effects, including improved functional capacity, neuronal connections and reduced anxiety [80]. Similar experiments conducted with transgenic mice found that an enriched environment compared with an impoverished environment reduces psychological stress, and strongly modulates the generation of Aβ (beta amyloid peptides) in vivo and its impact on the nervous system in animals with Alzheimer's disease [81]. Conversely, exposure to an impoverished environment has been found to lead to delayed brain maturation [82] and cognitive dysfunction in animals [83]. The concept of environmental enrichment has only seldom been transposed to humans, no doubt because of the technical and ethical complexity of conducting such experimental studies [84] However, many studies in the scientific literature assess the relationship between hospital environments and human health. It is critical to understand how existing research conducted in nursing homes might help in designing the ideal environment with evidence of benefits for the residents' health and well-being [85-86] . A systematic literature review of scientific studies examining the association between environmental factors and the health and well-being of individuals in the specific context of nursing homes provides an interesting report of the current knowledge, practices and efforts in modelling the physical environment in favour of the health and well-being of nursing home residents. We searched major scientific databases (PubMed/MEDLINE and the Cochrane Library) using a dedicated search equation[6] and using state of the art methodology to select articles.

Selected articles met the following inclusion criteria:

- Articles in English
- Studies of older people in long-term care facilities
- Investigate associations between components of the physical environment and resident outcomes including measures of health or well-being. The physical environment describes both architectural features and sensory aspects of long-term care facilities. Health outcomes are related to health markers of a geriatric syndrome.

---

[6] ("Nursing Homes"[Mesh] OR "Homes for the Aged"[Mesh] OR "Assisted Living Facilities"[Mesh] OR "Long-Term Facility") AND ("Architecture"[Mesh] OR "Environment Design"[Mesh] OR "Health Facility Environment"[Mesh] OR (Physical AND Environment)) AND ("Aged"[Mesh] OR "Aged, 80 and over"[Mesh] OR ((older OR elderly) AND (people OR person OR patient OR resident))).

- Reporting original observational or interventional studies.

This scoping review [87] resulted with 59 articles meeting these criteria. Of the articles included, the first dates back to 1998 and 41 were published after 2010, reflecting the growing interest in this topic over the last decade. Studies were conducted in health care, gerontology and architectural engineering research laboratories throughout many countries around the world; but mostly in North America (USA n=22 and Canada n=7), Western Europe (Germany, UK, France, Scandinavia and Netherlands n=23) and the rest of the world (Australia n=5, Asia n=2, Israel n=1). Overall, the 59 studies included 1,389 nursing homes and 14,795 residents. The number of nursing homes per study ranged from one to 320, the number of residents per study varied from 14 to 4,205. Thirty-five studies (59.3%) were conducted with residents living with various stages of dementia. This overview highlights the wide variety of approaches used in these studies. While the previously mentioned studies on environmental enrichment had a fairly well-defined framework, those on the physical environment of geriatric institutions were conducted in very different contexts.

As the selected articles covered a wide range of physical environments, we classified them according to their specific field of investigation, forming five categories as follows:

1. Dining environment
2. Outdoor gardens
3. Sensory environment
4. Small-scale vs large-scale nursing homes
5. Other environmental features

Similarly, the methodologies used in these studies were not very consistent. We identified 18 interventional studies (including 6 randomised controlled trials), 40 observational studies including cross-sectional studies, longitudinal cohort studies, mixed methods studies, and one survey study. Some interventional and observational studies compared two or more types of environment. The others used an alternative methodological approach of investigating associations between environmental characteristics and resident outcomes.

An extremely wide variety of outcomes were collected employing an extremely wide variety of measurement tools. The diversity of evaluation tools employed underlines the difficulty of consolidating results or even conducting a meta-analysis. Some studies focused on behavioural problems such as the average number of disruptive behaviours, wandering patients, and agitation. Many studies evaluated cognition. Some studies focused on depression symptoms or looked at independence or quality of life. Articles evaluating the quality of sleep used sleep and daytime activity levels, while those assessing the dining environment measured energy and food intake, Body Mass Index, and eating behaviour. The risk of falling was measured by recording either the number of falls or using scales for predicting falls, such as the Unipodal stance and the Timed Up and Go. Other studies evaluated social interaction and engagement in activities.

This great diversity of research settings, methodologies and outcome measures has not facilitated the emergence of a clear vision of the ideal physical environment for nursing home residents. To date, despite the prolific resources deployed, there are no clear, science-based recommendations at either a European or global level that are likely to enhance quality of life, well-being and health for nursing home residents. Below is a summary of the main conclusions that have emerged from this analysis of the existing scientific literature.

3.1. Dining Room Environment

A number of factors expose older adults living in institutions, particularly those with cognitive disorders, to a high risk of weight loss and malnutrition. Numerous studies have reported the role of the physical environment as a critical factor influencing nutrition and social interactions among residents in long term care facilities. Experiments report different trends in the design of the dining environment. Some value the concept of a small dining room, which reduces stress and haste; another study valorises that home likeness was significantly associated with higher food intake [88]. It is therefore critical to have a summary of existing studies to identify what really contributes to better nutrition and socialisation.

Seven studies conducted in 73 nursing homes involving 1,995 residents examined the connections between the design of the dining environment and the residents' eating experience and nutrition. All seven studies showed significant connections between the environment and food intake or changes in body mass index. Home likeness, temperature, lighting, food volume, and traditional tray service or not are key parameters that influence the dining experience and suggest that fine-tuning dining rooms can have a positive influence on the nutrition of nursing homes residents. However, some key findings can be highlighted as follows:

- The home likeness of the environment is significantly associated with greater food intake
- Bulk catering encourages greater food consumption [89]
- Dining room renovation improved body weight (+2 kg after 6 months) and dining experience [90]
- A supportive environment (sensory stimulation) reduces eating disabilities [91]

While it is difficult to draw any conclusions from these studies about the ideal design of catering areas to encourage mealtimes and social interaction, it is clear that the physical environment has a major influence on the quality of a person's eating experience.

3.2. Garden & Outdoor Facilities

Although there are a large number of studies on the garden and the health of older adults, only eight of them met the inclusion criteria. Eight studies in 480 nursing homes involving 1,404 residents examined associations between gardens or access to outdoor facilities and various health outcomes. Gardens are generally described as a friendly environment for nursing homes residents, with seven of the eight studies reporting significant links between design characteristics and the residents' cognition, independence and disruptive behaviour. Most studies assessed the benefits of gardens by comparing groups of residents who did and did not visit gardens. One intervention study examined two different types of gardens, enriched or conventional [92]. It found significant benefits on cognition, independence and reduced risk of falls for participants encouraged to visit enriched gardens, while no significant effects were found in participants who were encouraged to visit conventional gardens. The observational studies all concluded that there was a significant link between garden attendance and a reduction in behavioural problems [93-94].

We will discuss in more detail the interventional and observational studies which have attempted to assess the effects of gardens on the health of residents. However, this literature review has revealed a number of methodological shortcomings in studies on institutional gardens. Gardens seem to be appreciated by residents and their families for the breathing space they offer in relation to the highly standardised architecture of geriatric institutions; so much so that gardens seem to be valued not for what they obviously offer, but for the difference they present from the residents' ordinary environment.

3.3. Sensory Environment

Sensoriality is undoubtedly the key concept for designating the stimulation produced by the environment on individuals. This sensory stimulation is either positive when it is correctly adapted (e.g., a pleasant fragrance) and of appropriate intensity, or negative, when it becomes a nuisance, if it is unpleasant (e.g., a bad smell) and/or of excessive intensity. The sensory environment depends, of course, on whether or not people perceive it, depending on their personal sensitivities and abilities, whether they are auditory, visual, olfactory, gustatory or tactile.

Sensory stimulation has gained in popularity in nursing homes and appears to be a very promising approach to improving mood disorders and behavioural problems. However, at present, supporting evidence for its effectiveness is fragmentary and contradictory.

Fifteen studies conducted in 81 healthcare facilities involving 886 residents examined the connections between the sensory environment and various health outcomes. Seven studies investigated the influence of different sensory stimuli (natural or artificial lighting, noise, smell, temperature and music) on depressive symptoms, engagement in activities, apathy, quality of sleep, circadian rhythm, and disruptive behaviour. Three studies focused on the effects of attending a multi-sensory room on behavioural problems. Six studies reported significant associations between sensory stimulation and one or more health factors.

As we shall see below, it is not easy to demonstrate the real effectiveness of sensory stimulation. There are many reasons for this difficulty. Of course, as we explained earlier, the study methodology is certainly a limiting factor, but it is not the only one. In the course of our work, we have come to realise that an individual's ability to perceive a sensory environment depends on a number of factors: the nature and intensity of the stimulation, of course; perceptive abilities, which vary from person to person and change with age; the individual's personal history, which has made them more or less sensitive to certain sounds, smells, lights, tastes, etc.; and also, the way in which they are inclined to interact with the environment. This inclination to interact with the physical environment is constructed precisely by the environment itself. It will therefore be interesting to discover, beyond existing scientific studies, how it is possible to facilitate or restore these environmental interactions.

3.3.1. Light
Nine studies aimed to optimally assess differences in artificial lighting or sunlight exposure by adjusting the intensity and colour of the light or by recording its current brightness. Three studies investigated the effects of artificial lighting while two other studies examined the effects of natural lighting on sleep and engagement in activities. High intensity bluish light was shown to significantly improve circadian rhythmicity and restless behaviour. Three other studies conducted in two nursing homes in Oregon and North Carolina, employed a similar protocol to evaluate the impact of different light exposure (2000-3000 lux vs 500 lux) on agitation in dementia, depression and daytime sleepiness [95-96]. The results indicated positive links between these human factors and specific light-tuning over the course of the day, with more significant associations between lighting and these factors for study participants experiencing severe dementia. Riemersma-van der Lek, Swaab and Twisk [97]and Sumaya [98] respectively reported in two randomised controlled trials a significant connection between the combination of light and melatonin and reduced disruptive behaviour, and 10 000 lux light exposure with reduced depressive symptoms ($p<0.01$). Natural light generally was found to be associated with greater daytime activity while artificial lighting has not generally shown significant associations with sleep quality. Light as a sensory environmental factor repeatedly shows significant connections with a reduction of disruptive behaviour (agitation), quantity of food in-take, circadian rhythm, and reduced apathy.

3.3.2. Fragrance
At a time when more emphasis is being placed on diffusing pleasant fragrances into the air, and when aromatherapy is taking on a more prominent role in non-medicinal practices, it is interesting to analyse the results of scientific studies conducted in this field. The first thing to note is that there are very few of them. This is probably due in part to the technical and logistical difficulties involved in carrying them out. Our systematic review of the literature identified only one valid study. Bae and Abimbolz [99] employed an interventional RCT method to explore the effect on depression of a lavender

scent in the air. The authors found no significant difference between the intervention and control group.

3.3.3. Noise and Sound

Sound stimulation, like olfactory stimulation, is particularly dependent on the type of sound. Language makes a very clear distinction on this point, since we refer to an auditory stimulus as a noise when it is a nuisance and we call it a sound or even a melody when it is a positive stimulus. We move into yet another dimension if a sound becomes music.

Three studies, all observational [100, 101, 102] investigated the association between environmental noise in nursing homes and the well-being of nursing homes residents. The main hypotheses concerned the effect of reducing noise interference on residents' calmness, sleep disturbance, and engagement in activities. The studies assessed the effect of different potential sources of noise pollution with various negative effects. The recommendations of the studies were to eliminate noise sources as much as possible.

Health professionals seem to agree that music can influence the body, mind and soul. In a sense, this convergence mirrors the universal precepts of life described by the classical views of music and medicine; moreover, these basic assumptions have been progressively studied with scientific methods. It is reported that scientists are increasingly recognising the ability of music to elicit physiological and cognitive responses, and to elicit and evoke images and associations that seem to be unique to each human being. In addition, music appears to enhance or diminish symptoms when used in combination with other treatment methods. Musical intervention in the medical environment aims to facilitate the treatment process, reduce stress and improve well-being, and essentially involves pre-recorded music for patients. A Swiss study [103] published in 2020 presents the evaluation of a musical intervention in nursing homes. In its conclusions, the authors suggest that: *"The residents reported mainly positive effects, which can be explained by the fact that the programme offered them, in an environment where they sometimes lacked novelty, a combination of receptiveness and activity on a subject they considered important. Thanks to music's ability to trigger memories and strengthen links with identity and biography, participation in the programme was a valuable opportunity for the residents to stimulate and improve their cognitive abilities. In addition, the collective dimension of the programme facilitated interpersonal relationships. This seems particularly important given the sense of isolation that respondents often feel in the context of nursing homes."*

This experiment highlights the paradoxical dimension of sensory stimulation such as music. It calls forth a sense of novelty in the environment, while at the same time appealing to the personal sensibilities of each individual. A Swedish study [104] reinforces this perception by highlighting the extent to which individual history and musical upbringing play an essential role. Added to this are differences in auditory perception, particularly among the older adults. It is well known that as people age, social interaction is reduced in the presence of sound, whatever the form of sound.

3.3.4. Multi-Sensory Rooms and Multi-Sensory Environment
Three studies on multi-sensory rooms found no significant association between the use of multi-sensory rooms and residents' mood, behaviour, and fall risk. One qualitative observational study assessed the effects of sensory stimuli such as sound, music, and light on disruptive behaviours, ranking the impact of these factors according to their impact on disruptive behaviours. In their study, Cohen-Mansfield [102] recorded the sensory parameters of noise, temperature, and light, and found significant effects on mood and engagement in activities.

Snoezelen rooms in nursing homes are regularly mentioned among the multi-sensory environments available. The studies identified in our literature review do not show any significant effect of their use [105]. Above and beyond the effective marketing approach used to promote them, it would seem that the main advantage of these Snoezelen rooms is that they allow residents to benefit from the support of a healthcare professional when they go there. And it is undoubtedly this time spent with them that has been most beneficial.

3.4. Small- vs Large-Scale Nursing Homes

For several decades now, there has been a tendency to consider that smaller nursing homes, designed around the concept of a "maisonette," and based on a residential approach, are much more conducive to the residents' quality of life. The Alzheimer's villages that have been experimented with since 2009 in a number of Western countries are largely based on this concept. The Green House project we described above is very much in line with this philosophy. This initiative, which is regularly taken up by architects and health authorities, deserves to be evaluated using a scientific approach that compares the architectural dimension with the health and quality of life of residents.

Our study compiles eleven studies involving 114 nursing homes and 2,165 residents, comparing the health of residents in small and/or family-type nursing homes with that of residents in large traditional institutions. The studies evaluate and compare health or Quality of Life outcomes of residents living in different size-scale facilities. Seven of these studies focused on residents living with dementia. De Boer , Beerens and Katterbach [106] observed, after subjecting Dutch residents to a dementia assessment tool, that small-scale, homelike nursing homes did not show significant differences with residents living in traditional large-scale nursing homes. Furthermore, McFadden [107] observed potential behaviour changes after residents relocated to a small-scale nursing home from a traditional one and did not find any association between relocation and behavioural improvement. Another study reported by Palm [108] in Germany, could not demonstrate differences in quality of life (using a dedicated QoL scale) between small- and large-scale units. However, it is difficult to assess the extent to which design factors relate to the residents' quality of life and behavioural problems. The results do not show a consistent effect of small-sise establishments on improving outcomes - five studies show no significant correlation between the size of the nursing home and the residents' health, while five studies conclude that small nursing homes have a positive effect on the activity levels of their residents.

These unexpected results seem to call into question the trend towards small is beautiful. It does, however, suggest that there are environmental factors other than the simple notion of size involved in responding to the health needs of frail people. Ultimately, whether the environment is more or less sensory, and whether the institution is larger or smaller, these studies reveal that it is not only the architectural design that is at stake, but also the opportunities for residents to develop interactions that are not simply passive.

3.5. Other Design Features of Nursing Homes

As we have seen, these legitimate efforts by institutions to design a health-friendly environment have often required substantial technical and financial resources. Our literature review enabled us to isolate a large number of studies which have shown significant results after having implemented sometimes minor changes in the living environment of the participating residents.

Twenty-one studies in 641 nursing homes, involving 8,345 residents, examine connections between other design features and various health outcomes. In one study a sky-like ceiling and lighting changes in shared spaces and corridors were found to significantly reduce wandering, shouting and agitation/aggression. Home likeness and shorter corridor length were significantly related to improved quality of life, reduced disruptive behaviour, and increased social interactions. In another interventional study, hallways in which benches and coffee tables, wall posters, artificial plants, and olfactory stimuli were added, resulted in reduced behavioural problems. Chenoweth, Forbes and Fleming [109] hypothesized that the installation of a person-centred care environment (PCE) would achieve similar outcomes to person-centred care (PCC) itself, for which they had already shown evidence of positive effects. They observed that PCE showed a significant reduction in agitation. Simpson, Lamb and Robert [110] evaluated the risk of hip fracture correlated with different types of flooring and identified that the lowest fall risk occurred on wood-carpeted floor. In Taiwan, Chang, Li and Porock [111] evaluated the potential effects on the well-being of residents living with dementia by decorating four floors of a nursing home with different themes. The links Chang found were related to reductions in agitation, orientation, fall risk, disorientation, activity participation, well-being, and depressive symptoms. Individually, each of the papers in this section identifies significant or non-significant associations between particular architectural parameters and the living and health conditions of nursing homes residents.

In this scoping review, we found numerous studies that examine connections between the physical environment of nursing homes and the residents' health. Most of the studies concluded that particular environmental features had a positive influence on outcomes for the residents. It should be noted that five interventional studies, particularly one randomised controlled trial clearly showed benefits for the residents' health or well-being.

The main lessons learned from the articles we analysed, were the descriptions of the impact of architectural features at all levels. One lesson is that each level and each component potentially have a specific impact, and therefore each environmental component needs to be considered carefully for its potential impact on the health of nursing home residents.

While we can identify the research-based impacts on the residents' health as described in many of the articles we analysed, the conclusions drawn in one nursing home are often not confirmed in another. Many of the favourable environmental characteristics that we identified are relatively easy to implement. This includes adjusting artificial lighting in different spaces, increasing exposure to natural light, and reducing noise pollution. Resident-focused interior renovations can make a valuable contribution to reducing behavioural problems. For example, an adapted dining-room layout, for the benefit of well-being and improved food-intake can be imagined without necessarily committing a high budget. However, the widely-held view that reducing the scale of nursing homes can contribute positively to quality of life was not formally confirmed by the research in the selected articles of our literature review. Some studies confirmed the value of small units, while several studies showed no significant difference for residents' health outcomes between small and large units.

The effect of the physical environment of nursing homes on residents living with dementia was extensively investigated. It is well recognised that cognitively impaired residents require specific adaptations to their living environment. Such studies, to be valid and reliable, require that we take into account the residents' frailty: for example, a resident's hearing ability will likely modulate the benefits of noise reduction on apathy. Low, Draper and Brodaty [112], Morgan-Brown, Newton and Ormerod [113], Marquardt [58], and Nordin, McKee K and Wallinder [114], highlight that dementia-friendly environments for persons living with dementia tend to be those specifically designed to promote independence and support well-being. The research from these authors highlights that the benefits of a dementia-friendly environment depend on the severity of dementia. Additionally, some of the selected articles make the point that the physical environment interacts with the cultural and social environment. This relationship is complex as Innes, Kelly and Dincarslan [115] and Low [112] concluded. These authors make the point that environmental design cannot be adjusted to the expectations of all residents *"some will need more security, while others will need more freedom to move around; some will prefer single rooms while others will prefer the company of shared rooms."* This is also what de Rooij, Luijkx KG and Schaafsma [116] noted when comparing Dutch and Belgian nursing homes. Although the two countries are culturally and geographically close, significant differences emerged when comparing the physical environment with the residents' quality of life. Tao [117] presents a detailed assessment of the relationship between the length and height of partitions and the health status of nursing residents in Hong Kong. Clearly, what is valid in Hong Kong may not be consistent with European or North American culture.

In the articles we selected, most authors recognised the complexity of designing an appropriate evaluation methodology: defining and implementing research protocols that take account of all parameters involved - both environmental and health parameters. The diversity of study designs and assessment tools reflects this complexity, as well as the small number of randomised controlled trials (n=6). Intervention studies are interesting research designs to provide practical directions to optimise nursing home environments, but randomisation and researcher blinding– the gold standard for such studies – are technically difficult due to the object of research.

The potential adverse effects on the environment are also instructive. Cohen-Mansfield's study of 320 American care homes [118], found that restrained access to gardens was significantly linked to an increase in agitated behaviour. Marquardt [58] and Hill, Nguyen TH and Shaha [119] highlighted the number of barriers and the poor design of circulation systems (long, uniform corridors with low-intensity artificial lighting) as having a negative influence on residents' sense of direction and on the risk of falls. Garcia, Hébert M and Kozak [101] supported the idea that reducing ambient noise levels is associated with a reduction in disruptive behaviour.

This scoping review helps identify poor design practices that negatively affect residents. It also highlights the results of studies that fail to confirm accepted hypotheses, such as the effect of lavender scent aromatherapy, or a sensory garden, which failed to perform better than its control group.

The contribution of the physical environment to the health and well-being of frail people is a highly challenging issue to analyse. There are many contributing factors, and the methodologies used to analyse them may produce very different results depending on the case. For example, a qualitative study carried out with a group of residents immediately after the performance of a musical group asking them for their opinion will produce very different results from a quantitative assessment of behavioural disorders using a scale such as the Neuropsychiatric Inventory (NPI) carried out 15 days after the performance.

In addition to this methodological dimension, there is the social construction that governs the way we look at the environment. This social construction can contribute to a bias in observation. Music and gardens, for example, generally evoke a positive image. This suggestion is likely to produce a positive reaction from participants, regardless of the effects or not of the environment on their health markers.

This review of the scientific literature on the environment and health of people living in geriatric institutions has made an important contribution to our thinking. It has enabled us to put into perspective the different areas of health on which the physical environment can have an influence, with a population whose fragility and potential multiplicity of disorders and chronic pathologies are well-known. Envisioning the design of an environment that can respond to all or some of these health issues is, as we described in the introduction, a major challenge. While these interventional and observational studies have confirmed that the environment can play a key role, there is still a need to understand how this occurs and the areas in which it can have an impact. This must be done in a way that is free from the social constructs and unique characteristics of each individual.

Chapter 4

The Enriched Environment Concept

1. The Development of Enriched Environment

The enriched environment was first described in 1946 by Hebb [34] of McGill University (Montreal). This neuropsychologist observed that mice raised as pets solved problems and exercises better than mice raised in cages. In particular, he pointed out that the effects on their cognitive abilities when they reached adulthood were more marked when the mice were exposed to a favourable environment during the first 3 weeks of life, compared with exposure to the same environment for adult mice. As a neuropsychologist, Hebb was passionate about understanding the behavioural responses of animals subjected to more or less stimulating environments. In Hebb's work, the enrichment of the environment varied according to the study, ranging from living in a group with other conspecifics, to specific sensory stimulation associated with light and odours, as well as more or less complex exercises to obtain water or food. It was later, particularly in the 1960s, with the American research team of Bennett, Diamond, Krech & Rosenzweig [120], that the notion of an enriched environment revealed its potential.

By comparing different types of environment, some impoverished, others enriched, repeated experiments have established a correspondence between environmental enrichment (EE) and the volume and thickness of the cerebral cortex. One of the flagship experiments conducted by the team at the US National Institute of Mental Health [121] compared a group of rats exposed for a month to what they called a complex and stimulating environment (CSE) with another group of rats placed in isolation (IC). Exposure was programmed for a sequence of 30 minutes each day for the ECS group, in a space that stimulated cognitive functions and where sweet kibbles were distributed for each success in solving a problem. The composition of this space was changed each day. Meanwhile, the rats in the IC group remained in individual cages with 5 closed sides and a wire mesh front, thus achieving tactile and visual isolation, and their access to food and water was not restricted. This study, published by Diamond, Krech D and Rosenzweig in 1964, was entitled "The effect of an enriched environment on the histology of the cerebral cortex of rats."

The average thickness of the visual zone of the cerebral cortex of rats placed in an enriched environment was significantly greater (6.2% thicker) than that of rats placed in isolation, resulting in a 19% increase in the volume of the visual zone of the cerebral cortex for rats exposed to the enriched environment. The findings of Diamond represented a break with the previous assumption that the weight and structure of the brain were stable and insensitive to any form of environmental influence. The fact that exposure to an enriched environment contributed to modifying the size and structure of the rat brain opened up a world that was subsequently explored by numerous teams of neurobiologists and sociologists (Figure 5). This work, along with that of Hebb, was the starting point for a great deal of research into the concept of environmental enrichment.

Most of the studies conducted on this subject have been carried out on the murine model, an experimental model of laboratory mice used for scientific studies. A few studies have been carried out with other animal species such as chimpanzees or fish. The research teams therefore set out to identify the link that could be formed between the complexity of the environment and the learning capacity or memory of the animals.

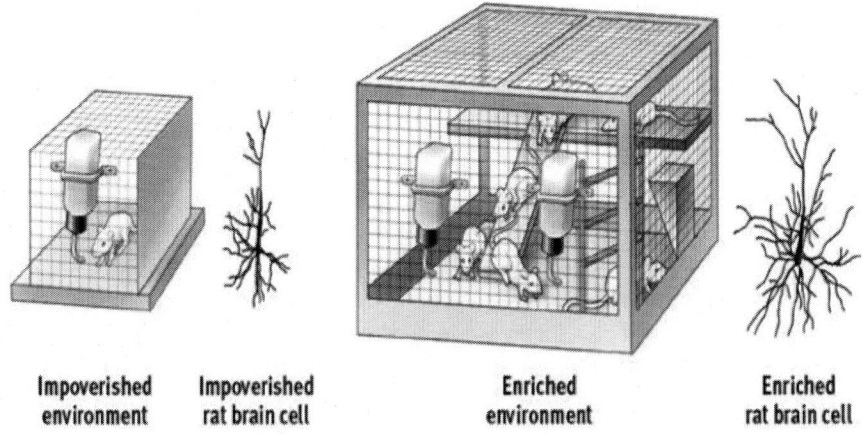

Figure 5. Effect of exposure to an enriched environment on neuronal ramification-Rosenzweig (1984).

Experiments carried out by Rampon, Jiang and Dong [122] at Princeton University showed that mice presented with unusual objects showed greater curiosity, abandoning ordinary objects. Measuring the mice's ability to memorise opened up a field of exploration into possible physiological changes linked to the environment. In particular, Rampon's team carried out a study on mice carrying a mutation in the gene coding for the NMDA glutamate receptor in the hippocampus, a mutation that is responsible for memory disorders in these animals. After repeated exposure to an enriched environment (EE), these mice carrying the mutation regained the same memory faculties as non-mutated mice.

The research carried out by various laboratories is forging a new understanding of the close link between the brain and the environment to which it is exposed. The fields of investigation are expanding:

- Yao, Zhang and Xie [123] showed in mice that EE prevents cognitive impairment and hyperphosphorylation of the Tau protein following chronic cerebral hypo-perfusion.
- A Japanese team [124] showed that EE compensated for memory deficits in mice carrying the PACAP -/- mutation, which disrupts neurotransmission, synaptic plasticity and neuronal survival.
- In 2005, Jankowsky, Melnikova and Fadale [81] studied transgenic mice over-expressing the ®-amyloid protein (one of the mouse models of Alzheimer's disease) and non-transgenic control mice (known as wild type), which were placed in enriched or standard cages at the age of 2 months and whose cognitive behaviour was tested after 6 months of differential housing. The EE made it possible to normalise the cognitive performance of the transgenic mice to the level of wild mice living in standard cages. Interestingly, these researchers showed that amyloid deposits in EE transgenic mice were comparable to those in transgenic mice reared in standard conditions, indicating that the favourable effects of EE occur despite the neuropathological process induced by this model. These results show that the effects of ®-amyloid deposits in vivo on nervous system function can be strongly modulated by environmental factors.
- Berardi, Braschi and Capsoni 2007 [125] also described the effects of EE on the progression of a mouse model of Alzheimer's disease observed in transgenic mice. Prolonged EE (2 to 7 months) significantly reduced the appearance of neuropathological signs of

Alzheimer's disease, and the authors concluded that EE slowed the pathological process in this mouse model.
- In 2005, Faherty, Raviie and Shepherd [126] published a study conducted on 3 groups of mice injected with a dose of 1-methyl-4-phenyl-1,2,3,6-tetrahydropyridine (MTPT - a classic model of experimental Parkinson's disease) and placed in environments described as 'enriched' (14 mice per cage equipped with moving wheels), 'exercise' (4 mice per cage also equipped with moving wheels) and 'standard' (4 to 6 mice per cage). The authors showed that the EE completely protected the mice in adulthood against the effects of Parkinson's disease induced by MTPT. In addition, they observed a 350% increase in the expression of glial cell-derived neurotrophic factor (GDNF), a growth factor strongly involved in brain plasticity, in mice with EE compared with unexposed mice.
- In 2016, the work of Mahati, Bhagya and Christofer [127] explored the effect of an enriched environment on severe depression induced in rats after injection of a toxic dose of clomipramine for 14 days. They observed a reduction in the expression of the depressive syndrome and anxiety for the EE group. In addition, EE reversed the volumetric alterations in brain areas that are observed in this experimental model of depression, particularly in the dentate gyrus and basolateral amygdala complex. Interestingly, in depressed rats subjected to EE, the volumes of these brain areas were significantly higher than in the control animals.
- Other studies published since 2010 have shown, in animal models, a positive effect of EE on sensations of chronic and inflammatory pain [120-122] and Rett syndrome [128].
- Numerous studies carried out to investigate EE have highlighted its effect on the development of social interactions in caged rodent populations, as well as on sleep in elderly mice [129].
- In 2017, Zarif, Nicolas S and Petit-Paitel [130] published a review article in which they analysed the various physiological processes by which EE induces a change in neuronal morphology, modifying synaptic plasticity and promoting angiogenesis (Figure 6).

Their conclusions are synthesised in the figure below.

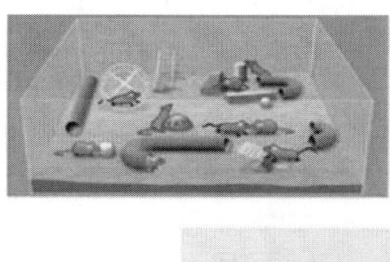

Enriched environment
- Sensory stimulations
- Physical activity
- Exploration, learning
- Social interactions

Endocrine systems
Hormones (corticosterone, NA)

Adipose tissue
Adipokines (leptin, adiponectin)

Afferent nerve endings upon muscle stimulation
Endorphins

Fluid circulation
Nutriment intake, Elimination of toxic metabolites

Immune systems
T cells..., cytokines, chemokines

Blood Brain Barrier
Choroid Plexus Barrier

Cerebral activity
Neurotrophic factors (BDNF, IGF1, VEGFα, NGF)

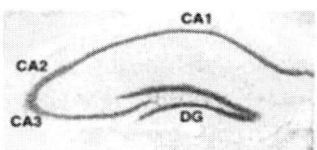

Hippocampus plasticity
- Neurogenesis in DG
- Synaptogenesis
- Synaptic plasticity
- Glia plasticity:
Oligodendrocytes (myelination)
Anti-inflammatory actions
(astrocytes and microglial cells)
- Angiogenesis

Figure 6. Enriched environments can modulate hippocampal plasticity via multiple pathways (Zarif 2017).

2. Enriched Environments Used in Experimental Work on the Murine Model

The methods used to enrich the environment varied greatly in the experimental studies we have reported. Rampon [122] working on the effect of EE on gene expression in the brain, described their model as follows: *"The enriched environment consisted of two large black plywood boxes containing various toys, wooden blocks, a pastry wheel and small houses. In the box, bottles of food and water were available to the animals. The mice were trained daily for 3 hours in each of the two boxes, the elements of which were changed or rearranged every half day."* The study by Rampon concluded that EE influences the expression of certain genes involved in neuronal structure, synaptic signalling and plasticity. Some of these genes are known to be associated with learning and memory. He, Tsipis and LaManna [131], in their study of the relationship between EE and brain capillary density and cognitive ability, used fairly similar equipment: *"The enrichment cages were provided with toys of different sises, shapes and textures, in order to promote visual and sensory stimulation and physical activity through climbing, burrowing and exploration. Toys were exchanged between enrichment cages approximately every three days for the duration of the study. Groups of three mice were housed in each enrichment cage to avoid overcrowding and competition. Non-enriched control mice were kept in standard housing without enrichment and were monitored at regular intervals."* Compared with the control group, the EE group had significantly higher capillary density (~30%) in the cortical brain.

As part of a Brazilian study on EE and anxiety, Kimura, Mattaraia and Picolo [132] described the equipment used as follows: *"The first EE model tested (simple EE) was introduced after weaning - the animals were placed in normal-sised cages with one of three different objects (cardboard tubes, plastic cylinders or disposable caps) introduced into the cage and changed each week by the other object in alternation, in order to maintain novelty. For the second EE protocol tested (enhanced EE), enrichment began at birth and consisted of adding various objects to the animals' cages. Each type of object was changed weekly. After 5 weeks, the animals were placed in larger cages than the standard cages, with five different types of object at a time, one of which was changed every week. Animals not subjected to EE were handled in the same way as the EE groups."*

A reading of the numerous publications on this subject highlights a few main points:

- A tendency to reuse enrichment methods that have given positive results in previous studies.
- An almost systematic practice of renewing the components of the enriched environment during the study period.
- An effort to modify the enrichment mode according to the therapeutic targets (cognitive disorders, inflammatory pain, Parkinson's disease, etc.).

However, it is difficult to extrapolate these practices to humans, but it is interesting to note a few ideas that are probably transferable, such as the diversity of stimulation modes, the presence of games and motivational elements, and the notion of renewing and changing stimulation modules.

3. Enriched Environment Studies on Humans

The idea that the environment can have an effect on human cognitive abilities was an accepted fact, supported in particular by the work of Van Alstyne [133] and then Gottfried [134]. This work presented the process of cognitive development in young children in relation to the influence of their family environment, based in particular on Piaget's measurements of sensorimotor abilities.

3.1. A Few Studies on Autism

The first studies evaluating the effects of EE in humans were carried out on people with Autism Spectrum Disorders (ASD). Particular mention should be made of the research by Woo [135], who suggests that the EE constitutes a therapeutic model for people suffering from ASD, and Sood [136], who envisages it as an educational programme to be adapted in schools catering for autistic children. In 2013, Woo, Donnelly and Steinberg-Epstein published a randomised controlled study involving 28 children with autism aged between 3 and 12 years, comparing the sensorimotor enrichment of the environment with changes in their cognitive abilities over a period of 6 months. In rats, environmental enrichment reversed many autism-like symptoms produced by prenatal exposure to valproic acid [137]. Enrichment normalised responses to sensory stimuli, induced stronger acoustic prepulse inhibition, decreased locomotor activity, reduced repetitive behaviour, increased exploratory behaviour, decreased anxiety and increased social interaction. The authors then suggested the use of environmental enrichment to treat the symptoms of autism in children. Similarly, after reviewing the literature describing the benefits of environmental enrichment for animal models of autism, Reynolds, Urruela and Devine [138] suggested that environmental enrichment could be beneficial for children with autism, noting that key aspects of environmental enrichment appear to include novel and diverse sensory experiences. To be included in the study, their combined communication and social interaction scores had to fall within the classification of autism, rather than the autism spectrum. Children with forms of autistic syndrome or childhood disintegrative disorder were excluded from the study. No psychotropic medication was administered throughout the study and anticonvulsants were only administered if the child had been on a stable dose for more than three months.

All children continued with their standard therapy. The combinations of various behavioural therapies used by the children are referred to as "standard care" and no statistically significant differences in the frequency of use of the therapies were observed between the groups. Children who met the inclusion criteria were randomly assigned to one of three groups. The first group consisted of control participants receiving usual care with only ongoing treatment. The full treatment group continued to receive their standard treatments, but in addition they received the full set of sensorimotor exercises [139], which activated different combinations of senses, including olfactory, tactile, thermal, auditory, visual and motor systems). The aim was also to determine whether a smaller set of exercises, with less novelty and requiring less parental time, would be as effective as the full set of exercises. A partial treatment group was therefore included, which received a subset of exercises excluding olfactory exercises, olfactory/tactile exercises and music. The parents of the children in both treatment groups received a kit containing the items needed for the sensorimotor exercises, as well as written instructions on how to use them.

After a short training session, the parents of both groups had their children complete four to seven exercises at home in the mornings and evenings. Each session lasted between 15 and 30 minutes in total, with some activities requiring additional preparation time. Every two weeks, the parents were contacted by e-mail and given a new set of exercises for their child; the exercises became increasingly difficult over the six months. The participants had a form of severe autism diagnosed at the start of the study and were divided into two groups: enriched with EE, and control without EE. The enriched group received sequenced sensory activities and interactions (sounds, colours, scents, temperature, etc.) and sensorimotor activity modules for the duration of the study. The results showed a significant improvement in the participants of the enriched group compared with the control group on 11 of the 15 evaluation criteria used, including emotional reaction, bodily ease, intellectual coherence of answers to questions, concentration, fear and nervousness. The effects obtained in this study were clearly superior to those obtained with other therapies used with autistic children. In 2015, the same authors published a complementary study [140] with a comparable and refined protocol. The results of this new study showed that after 6 months, the children in the enriched group showed a significant improvement in their intelligence quotient (IQ) score, a reduction in their atypical sensory reactions and an improvement in their language skills compared with the control group. In addition, 21% of the children in the enriched group no longer met the criteria for the severity of autism, although they remained on the autism spectrum. In their discussion, the authors suggest a future study to evaluate the level of enrichment needed to maintain or even improve these results over time.

Another study, reported by Sood, LaVesser P and Schranz [141], investigated the influence of the home physical environment on activities on children with ASD. Recent evidence suggests that parents of children with ASD report less participation by their children in the activities of daily life. For example, families of children with ASD aged 6 to 17 reported that their children participated less in after-school or weekend clubs or other organised events; they also participated less in community activities than families of typically developing children [142].

Physical and social environmental factors within the home can affect a child's development. Physical factors include the structure and density of the dwelling, the objects present in the dwelling, the quality and characteristics of the dwelling, the predictability of daily routines, residential mobility and the availability of resources.

The physical structure of a home can help children learn and acquire developmental skills if the environment is accessible. However, the physical environment can also impose barriers to participation; for example, lack of toys and equipment can limit exploration [143].

A child's social environment includes the people with whom they form relationships at home, at school and in the community. These may include family, peers and neighbours. As children grow and develop, their social environment changes. The family of a child with ASD plays an essential role in "determining the type and number of activities in which the child will have the opportunity to participate."

An exploratory correlational research model was used by Sood. The aim of a correlational study is "to explore the nature of existing relationships between variables" to explore the nature of existing relationships between variables"[144]. Using this study design, the researchers sought to identify and explore any relationship between parental stress, the quality of the family environment and the children's participation in family activities.

For this study, subscales were used to measure participation in domestic activities:

- Domestic activities: cooking, hanging up a coat, setting or clearing the table, sweeping, emptying the bins, fetching the mail, working in the yard, looking after a pet, cleaning, helping with the laundry and washing up.
- Low-demand leisure activities: building with blocks, playing with playdough, playing alone, playing on the computer, cutting out, doing puzzles, swinging, watching TV, listening to music, colouring and pretending.
- Social interaction activities include roughhousing, taking turns, reading books, cuddling, going for walks, talking on the phone, going to birthday parties, talking to friends, playing with children, visiting and getting together with family members.

A number of participants indicated that an organised and designated play area for a child within the home is crucial for the development of the child's motor, sensory, cognitive and social skills. Play areas should include developmentally appropriate (i.e., age-appropriate) toys and learning materials that can support the development of motor, sensory and social skills.

In addition, participants highlighted that disorganised and unstructured play areas for children and/or a lack of resources at home (e.g., toys, books, play equipment and games) can inhibit the participation of children with ASD in the home environment.

This study provides a beginning characterization of the environmental factors dedicated to cognitive, learning, social and emotional stimulation - that influence the participation of children with ASD in home activities. It may further inform occupational therapists about potential home environment factors that may facilitate or hinder the participation of children in their activities of daily life. It also emphasises the need to design appropriate assessment scales to evaluate the quality of environmental enrichment in the homes of children with ASD.

3.2. The Leipzig Study

A longitudinal study [145] was conducted in 2013 by researchers at the University of Leipzig to investigate the role of environmental factors and the risk of developing Alzheimer's disease. In a cohort of 903 participants aged 75 or over at the start of the study, exposure to certain environmental factors was recorded. The participants were followed for 8 years, with detailed cognitive assessments every 18 months. The aim was to assess the potentially protective role of an enriched environment on the prevalence of Alzheimer's disease. During the inclusion interviews, the exposure to an enriched environment during their working life was determined on the basis of 4 classification indices created for this study and inspired by the work on the EE carried out on mice: "*Novelty, Fluid, Verbal and Executive.*" *Novelty*: describing the frequency of new situations encountered in working life; *Fluid*: indicating cognitive stimulation on fluid intelligence; Verbal on crystallised intelligence; *Executive*: measuring the level of independence and task planning. The authors compared the initial characteristics of participants who had developed Alzheimer's disease during the follow-up period with those of people who had not.

The results showed a significant association between a high value of the 'Executive' index and a lower prevalence of Alzheimer's disease. While the Leipzig study does not allow us to conclude that there is a causal link between the EE and the incidence of Alzheimer's disease, it does open up an interesting avenue of investigation into the relationship between an enriched environment and the risk of Alzheimer's disease in humans.

4. The Enriched Environment Research: A Wealth of Knowledge

These enriched environment studies have been carried out for over 70 years in numerous laboratories, mainly neurobiology laboratories. They have accumulated a wealth of knowledge, exploring the different ways in which the environment can be enriched, the different pathologies that EE can treat, and also the mechanisms of action of EE on the cerebral cortex of mice.

Although originally described by Rosenzweig as a *"combination of inanimate and social stimulation"* [146], EE currently refers to "housing conditions that enhance sensory, cognitive, and motor stimulation." In an animal context, these conditions include larger cages, with several objects such as tunnels, stairs, hiding places, seesaws, and a wheel; which are changed periodically to stimulate curiosity and exploration. There are several protocols for EE, which vary in terms of the type of box cage, kind, and number of objects, and type of nest. Moreover, strain, age, and duration of EE exposure may affect the outcome. As to humans, changes in the environment usually include family, friendship, hobbies, socioeconomic status, and schooling among others, with EE being, therefore, characterised by the association of these elements. EE exposure is a promising strategy for the treatment of neurodegenerative diseases, as it can cause structural and functional changes in the brain, promoting neurogenesis and dendritic growth. It does so by inducing alterations in gene expression levels and by enhancing the expression of neurotrophic factors. In addition, it increases neurotransmission modulation and may influence the immune system.

A number of studies analysed the impact of EE at the molecular level on dopamine transporter (DAT) and investigated how this strategy affects the transport of monoamines in toxin-induced models of Parkinson disease [147]. DAT plays a key role in the initial events of MPTP toxicity, since the toxic metabolite MPP+ is a high-affinity substrate for this transporter demonstrated that a 2-month exposure to EE prevents the loss of dopamine neurons in the SNpc of MPTP-treated mice. In line with these results, it has been shown through densitometric analysis that EE downregulates the striatal levels of DAT mRNA and decreases the DAT-binding capacity in the rostral caudate-putamen of MPTP-treated mice when compared with animals exposed to a standard environment. Regarding DAT, it has been suggested that the protection elicited by EE may be mediated, at least in part, by increased levels of growth factors such as brain-derived neurotrophic factor (BDNF).

The effects of environmental enrichment on neurotransmitters such as dopamine, acetylcholine, serotonin, glutamate and noradrenaline have been described. Some are summarised in the Figures 7 to 10 below.

These figures selected from the thousands of studies carried out on enriched environments, contrast with the more approximate reading of the studies carried out in geriatric institutions. The highly standardised methodology and well-defined environmental framework enabled the research teams to produce results with evidential value. We have explored this scientific literature and present a summary here.

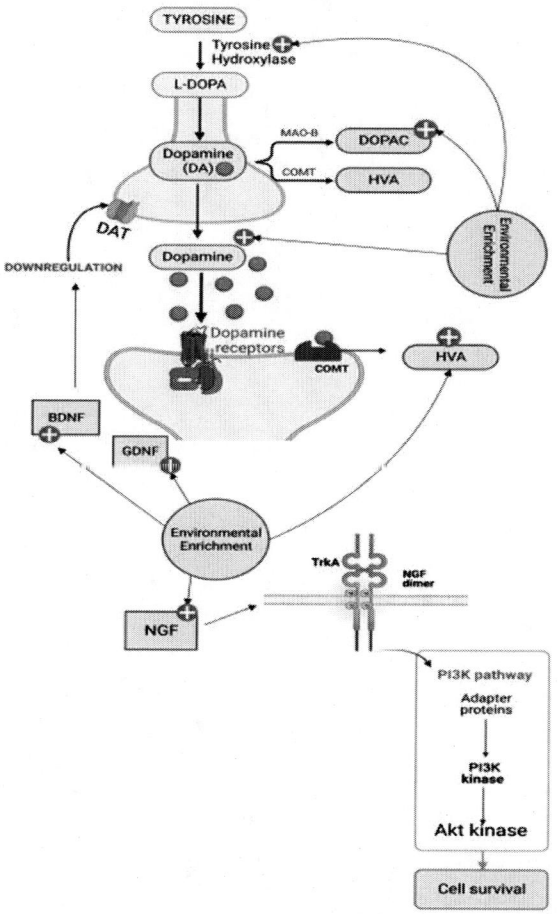

Figure 7. Effects of environmental enrichment on the dopaminergic system. Dopamine is synthesised from tyrosine by tyrosine hydroxylase into levodopa (L-DOPA) and then decarboxylated into dopamine. The effects of dopamine are mediated by dopamine receptors. To stop signalling, extracellular dopamine is either eliminated by neuronal reuptake via the dopamine transporter (DAT) or metabolised by monoamine oxidase B (MAO-B) and catechol-O-methyl transferase (COMT) to 3,4-dihydroxyphenylacetic acid (DOPAC) and homovanillic acid (HVA), respectively. Environmental enrichment increased tyrosine hydroxylase expression and DOPAC and HVA levels in DP models (positive sign). In addition, environmental enrichment downregulates DAT levels and decreases DAT binding by increasing brain-derived neurotrophic factor (BDNF) (positive sign). In addition, environmental enrichment increases glial-derived neurotrophic factor (GDNF) and nerve growth factor (NGF) (positive sign), which produces its effect via the PI3K pathway. produces its effect via the PI3K pathway. From Alarcon, Presti-Silva and Simões 2022 – Neural Regen Res. [147].

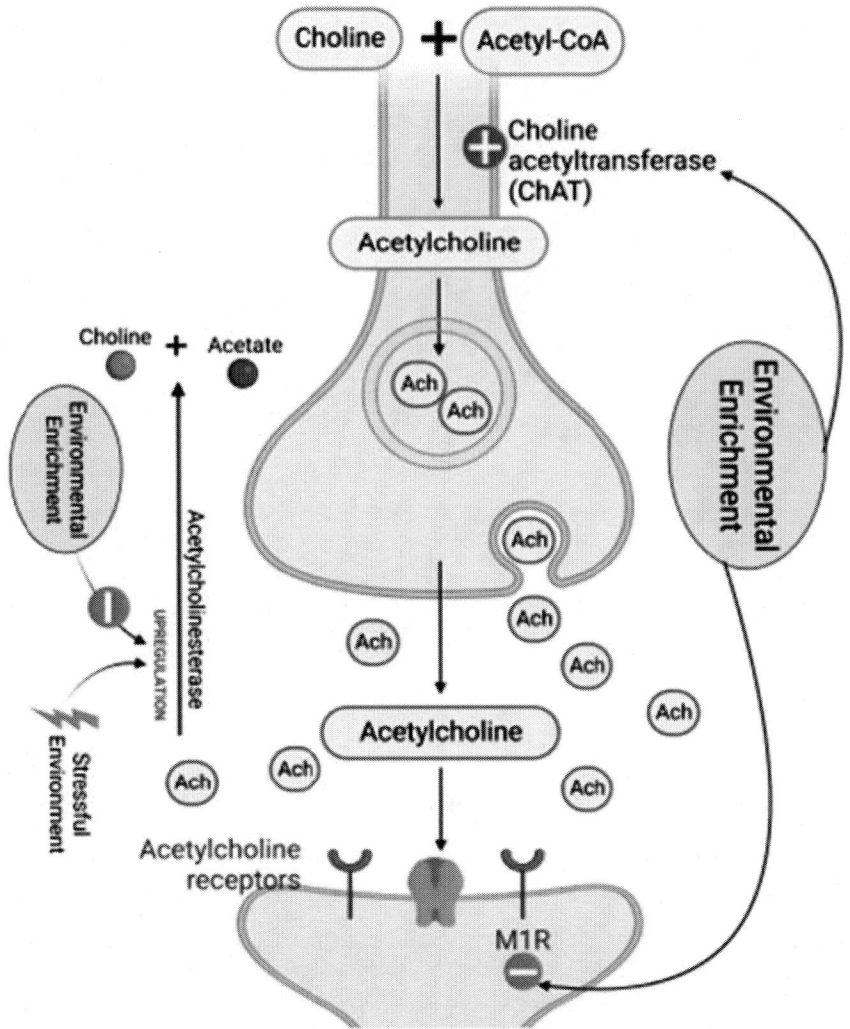

Figure 8. Effects of environmental enrichment on the cholinergic system. Acetylcholine (ACh) is synthesised in neurons from choline and acetyl-coenzyme A by the enzyme acetyltransferase (ChAT). ACh is loaded into synaptic vesicles and is released from nerve terminals. The effects of ACh are mediated by the activation of ionotropic or metabotropic receptors such as muscarinic ACh receptor (M1R). ACh is degraded into choline and acetate by the enzyme acetylcholinesterase. A stressful environment upregulates acetylcholinesterase enzyme and environmental enrichment downregulates it (minus sign). Also, environmental enrichment upregulates acetyltransferase enzyme expression (positive sign) and downregulates M1R expression. From Alarcon 2022 – Neural Regen Res [147].

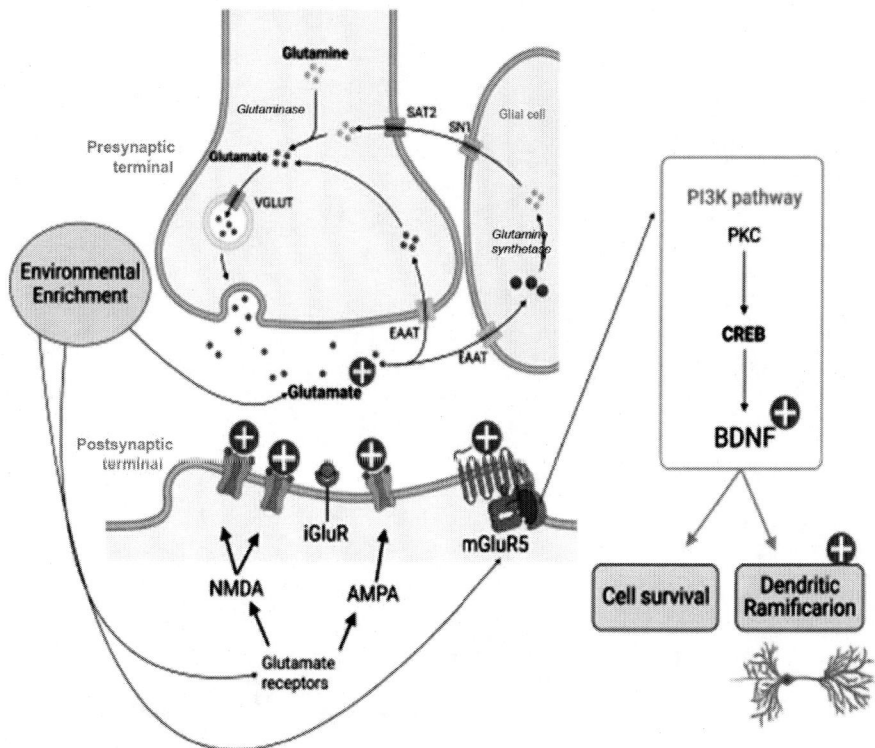

Figure 9. Effects of environmental enrichment on the glutamatergic system. Glutamate is synthesised from glutamine in a reaction catalyzed by glutaminase. Glutamate is then packaged into synaptic vesicles by the vesicular glutamate transporter (VGLUT) and released from nerve terminals. The effects of glutamate are mediated by the activation of ionotropic receptors (iGluR such as N-methyl-D-aspartate (NMDA) and a α amino3-hydroxy-5-methyl-4-isoxazolepropionic acid (AMPA) receptor) and metabotropic receptors such as mGlutamate is removed from the synapse by excitatory amino acid transporters (EAATs) present on glial cells and neighbouring neurons. Within the glial cell, glutamate is converted to glutamine by glutamine synthetase and glutamine is then released by the N transport system (SN1) and taken up by neurons by the A system (SAT2). Environmental enrichment increases basal glutamate levels and the expression of AMPA and NMDA (positive sign). In addition, it increases BDNF levels (Brain derived neurotrophic factors) and the expression of dendritic branches of pyramidal cells by activation of mGluR5 (positive sign). BDNF, CREB (cAMP- Response Element Binding Protein), PKC (Protein Kinase C). From Alarcon 2022 – Neural Regen Res [147].

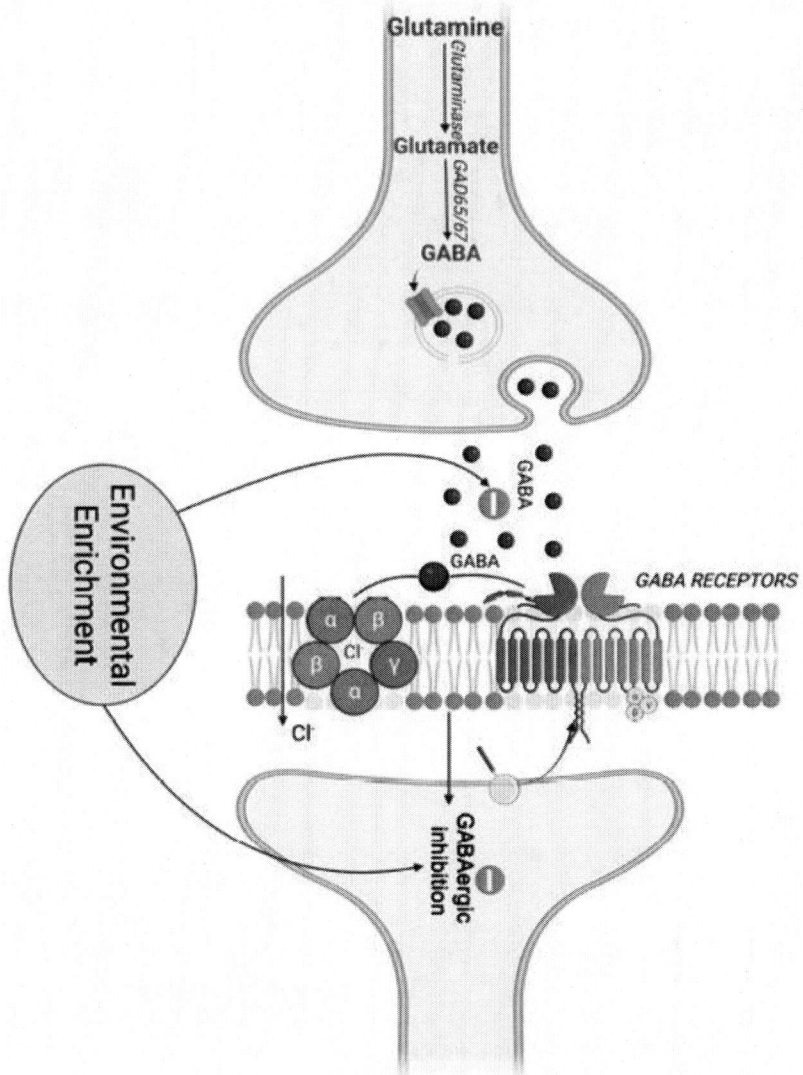

Figure 10. Effects of environmental enrichment on the GABAergic system. GABA is synthesised in the pre-synaptic terminal from glutamate by glutamic acid decarboxylase (GAD) enzymes, GAD65 and GAD67. GABA is loaded into synaptic vesicles by a vesicular neurotransmitter transporter and is released from nerve terminals. The effects of GABA are mediated by the activation of ionotropic or metabotropic receptors. Environmental enrichment downregulates basal GABA concentrations and GABAergic inhibition (minus sign). From Alarcon 2022 – Neural Regen Res [147].

Most of these studies were conducted on animal models (mainly mice, fish and chimpanzees), with the exception of few studies conducted on humans, in particular Alzheimer's disease and autism. Most of the studies we reviewed led the authors to conclude that the enriched environment had a significant and positive effect on the health criteria studied, including behaviour, anxiety, cognition and the expression of proteins specific to the functions studied. The fields explored by research into environmental enrichment are numerous. They use standardised experimental models, mainly on mice (or rats), to examine the effects of the environment on the many pathologies, stresses and disorders that an individual may suffer in the course of his or her life. They highlight the plasticity of the brain, which reacts by compensating for the cerebral zones affected, creating parallel information circuits.

The Figure 11 below summarises the different fields of investigation explored in recent decades.

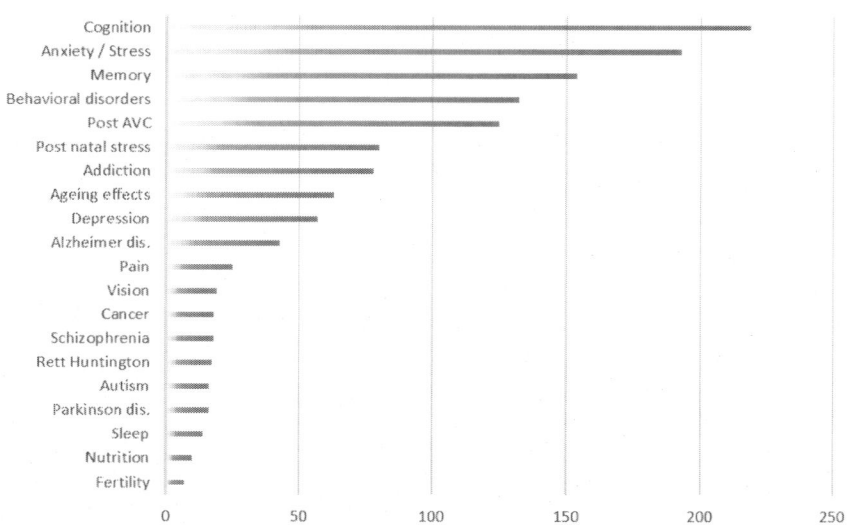

Figure 11. Number of inventoried scientific publications on environmental enrichment PubMed in Nov 2022.

This non-exhaustive survey of the literature provides an overview of the range of areas of interest covered by environmental enrichment and its potential for application to humans.

Chapter 5

Transposition of Environmental Enrichment to Humans

The transposition of the "enriched environment" concept to the experimental setting imposes a number of constraints in terms of methodology and purpose. Having chosen to transpose the concept to the environment of the older adults, for the reasons outlined above, the need to design a suitable enriched environment naturally led us to focus our studies on nursing homes. However, in France as elsewhere in the world, nursing homes are subject to numerous regulatory and normative constraints, which do not facilitate temporary modifications to the environment for the purposes of scientific studies. This is all the more true, given that the initial phases of the studies were designed to be exploratory in nature, in order to validate their transposability to humans. Of course, enriching the collective spaces within a nursing home was an interesting opportunity, given that their architecture often resembled an impoverished environment! What's more, the budgetary resources required for a pilot phase were too high to justify a one-off investment. This is why we quite naturally oriented our transposition project towards outdoor spaces in geriatric institutions, knowing that the financial requirements and normative constraints were far less significant there.

As we shall see, outdoor spaces, and in particular gardens, are well represented in nursing homes, and it seemed possible to develop the concept of the enriched garden by replicating it in several establishments in order to build multi-centre research protocols. Before going any further in describing the concept of the "enriched garden," we need to describe and understand the heritage and the social and cultural constructs that gardens carry, in order to identify the notions that gardens represent and to extract ourselves from them to avoid bias in our studies.

1. The Garden Experiences

Understanding the social construct of gardens suggests that they carry a heritage that has facilitated their designation as a health-promoting environment. From the very beginning, gardens have been part of the environment in which people live. Gardens have provided a physical representation of man's imaginary ideal. The idea of gardens has travelled through cultures and civilizations, receiving a variety of philosophical, religious, political, artistic and cultural influences. Gardens were created in their own location, with their individual architecture and choice of plant palette and materials. The Garden of Eden, the gardens of Babylon, mediaeval or Andalusian gardens, the gardens of Chinese scholars, royal gardens or English gardens... each of them demonstrates man's domination over nature in the service of an ideology, a school of thought, a religion or a political hold over a territory - Hildegarde Von Bingen combines this with the poetry inspired by the Hortus Conclusus in a representation of the Song of Songs:

"Hortus conclusus soror mea sponsa; hortus conclusus, fons signatus"
("My sister and betrothed is an enclosed garden; the enclosed garden is a closed spring").

This Hortus Conclusus, which in the Middle Ages became the space dedicated to the cult of the Virgin Mary, associated with a vision of paradise, is the vision that has travelled down to the present day when we speak of the mediaeval garden. Both the Catholic Church and Islam used the garden as a vehicle for representing their religious ideals. In addition to iconography, the garden was a popular medium for representing religious values and even paradise (pairidaēza means garden in Avestian Iranian). Nowadays, this codification of the world reduced to the space of a garden takes on an almost mystical, idealised dimension in a period that is itself in search of spirituality.

1.1. Hanging Gardens of Babylon

Their ruins have never been found, and yet the mere mention of the Hanging Gardens of Babylon is enough to conjure up a mythical fresco. This fresco highlights extraordinary hanging gardens made up of orchards and vegetable gardens, irrigated by endless screws using water drawn from the Euphrates. This vision of prosperity in an arid landscape, this projection of luxuriant harmony fit for a king, this flow of nature between earth and sky has fuelled many a fertile imagination.

The imaginary dimension associated with the hanging gardens of Babylon only reinforces their mythical nature. Representations of these gardens abound, derived from stories transcribed by the Greeks, and feeding the legend of King Nebuchadnezzar or the King of Nineveh. With no archaeological basis, these images trace the furrows of dreams and the boundaries of the possible. In Babylon, the hanging gardens make you dizzy, and are the source of the string of virtues that have adorned gardens over the centuries.

The general architecture of these gardens, the cultivation and watering techniques used and the plants grown there all suggest abundance and excess, opening the door to dreams.

Despite the relentless excavations carried out at the beginning of the 20th century on the archaeological site of Babylon, when the mythical buildings of the city were rediscovered, no trace of the hanging gardens has been found. And while further work may uncover what remains a mystery and an enigma today, it is important to remember that despite the absence of tangible evidence, the fairytale dimension of the hanging gardens of Babylon has never ceased to exist. The accounts of the ancients, which are difficult to verify, and many graphic representations continue to maintain the perception of an exceptional place... no doubt because people need this imaginary and grandiose representation of the gardens even more than the discovery of their archaeological remains.

1.2. Persian Gardens

The origins of Persian gardens (in Persian: باغ های ایرانی) are thought to date back to 4000 BC, but they really took off from the 11th century onwards, reaching their apogee in the 16th and 17th centuries. They remain emblematic of a vision of paradise, so much so that the Persian word for an enclosed space, in this case a garden, was "pairi-daeza" - terminology that has been passed down under the name of paradise.

The image of these gardens that has endured throughout history is one of precision and symmetry in the alignments, but also the splendour of the vegetation, the abundance of fruit and the richness of the ornate landscape.

They also stand out for the diversity and attention paid to expressing and stimulating the senses: the lights shimmering in glass crystals, the colours resonating with each other, the slender shapes of the cypress trees swaying in the wind, the fragrance of the flowers and the intoxicating taste of the wine... The emotions combine with the spirit in Persian gardens, inviting us to a spiritual recreation, before the encounter with paradise.

Persian gardens are part of this ideal vision of gardens in general. In Isfahan, the capital of the Persian Empire, water is a constant presence, through irrigation, playgrounds and ponds, thanks to the presence of a large river - the Zayandeh - and an artificial network that fertilises this region surrounded by desert. This vision of fertility in the middle of an arid land reinforces the image of gardens as an earthly ideal.

Persian gardens exist not just because of what they are, but also because of what people do in them. People pray in them, dream in them, and write poems in them. Hafiz, a 14th-century Persian poet whose mausoleum stands in the middle of the garden at Shiraz, was one of these lyrical poets. He wrote odes to the pleasures of life, often setting his poems in gardens.

A source of inspiration, a place of peace and lyricism, the Persian garden expresses the horizon of a hope for the world, in all the fields of the happy imagination, uniting life and death in a harmonious silhouette.

This is what people have wanted to give Persian gardens, this is how Persian gardens have survived the ages, and this is how we perceive them in such a sublime way, as painted in Hâfez poetry:

"Early in the morning I went to the garden to pick a rose.
    Suddenly the voice of a nightingale came to my ear

    The poor thing, like me, had fallen in love with a rose
    And his cry of distress caused a tumult in the flowerbed

    I turned in this flowerbed and this garden; from moment to moment
    I thought of this rose and this nightingale.

    The rose having become the companion of beauty, the nightingale the intimate of love
    In him no change, in the other no variation.

    When the voice of the nightingale made its mark on my heart,
    I changed so much that I had no patience left.

    In this garden so many roses bloom, but
    No one has plucked a rose without the scourge of the thorn.

Hâfez, of the world in its rotation does not hope for appeasement:
It has a thousand faults and has not one favour!"[7]

"Bring, O cupbearer, bring the rest of our wine, for you will not find in Paradise either this bank of Roukn Abad or the gardens of Goulguecht or Mousalla."[8]

1.3. Gardens of Chinese Scholars

The gardens of Chinese Scholars do not play with the imaginary, they are the imaginary [148]. They are the imagination of these idle rich Chinese who have withdrawn from the imperial court to devote themselves to their ideal. A life in harmony with nature, punctuated by the erudite pleasures of tea, wine, painting, poetry and gallantry. They can only be read and understood through dreams, imagination or travellers' accounts of the landscapes they encountered. These gardens bring the world together and represent it; they are the centre of gravity of the imagination, the projection of a vision of the world in a smaller world. Every particle of nature is domesticated by this human interpretation. Birds sing, but in a cage, fruit trees grow to form surprising sculptures directed by pruning, sand is smoothed, gravel is raked along precise cardinal lines, stone is arranged in a measured geometry, water spreads out in a pond to form a mirror to the stars, trees are mastered to the point of offering the dwarf shapes of bonsai creations. The fascination of these gardens lies in the distinction between visible and invisible landscapes.

For the Chinese Scholars, the garden enabled man to rediscover his centre of gravity, to extend his emotions and sensations in a reassuring, welcoming and understanding environment.

Nor can the gardens of the Scholars be detached from the way they are depicted. We see this in Chinese painting and the works codifying this painting (You shan, you shui 有山有水 - with mountains and water - a literal translation for a scenic and lyrical representation of a nature that cannot be described because it is intimately allied to the imaginary). This is particularly true of Wang Kai - a 17th-century Chinese painter - who wrote an educational

---

[7] From Hâfez (Khouajeh Chams ad-Din Mohammad Hafez-e Chirazi) - The rose, the nightingale and the poet in the garden (Ghazal 456).
[8] From Hâfez - River and Gardens of Shiraz - (Odes by Hafiz - Elzevirian Oriental Library, LVXXIIIp.i-xi).

work describing how nature should be represented (The Method of Painting the Mustard Seed Garden 芥子园) [149].

The composition and meticulous organization of these scholarly gardens are balanced between choices to conceal or show the vegetation, the profiles, the shapes, the depths, the horizon and the effect of passing time.

The images produced reflect the meanderings of the mind and suggest a link with the quest we make for ourselves. This quest resonates with the shadows, lights and contrasts that make up human nature. Implicit in the garden of the learned are so many milestones of the gardener's personality, contributing to a better understanding of oneself. The garden reveals man's nature and justifies his existential roots.

1.4. The Japanese Gardens on Kyushu Island

This exceptional relationship between man and his environment was also magnified by Japanese monks in the 12th century when they created the first tea gardens [150]. The Chinese influence was certainly not foreign to the structure and spirit of these gardens, but they found their uniqueness in Japan. The monks on the island of Kyushu used their gardens to demonstrate their capacity for meditation, a meditation they owe to their spirituality and philosophy. Their gardens had to reflect more than just their use: they had to be a concrete demonstration of an ideology - Zen Buddhism was at the heart of the power struggles in the Emperor's entourage - which meant that these gardens were a power issue. In Japan, as elsewhere, the garden is the vehicle for traditions handed down through the ages - rigorously combining precise architectural rules with cultural practices. In Kyushu, the garden is a benevolent setting for the home, and, as in China, a representation of the universe in all its details. The symbolism of the garden takes advantage of the perspectives of depth to convey messages to the visitor. The large Kyushu stones positioned in front of the smaller ones reinforce this illusion of eternity, to which the eye effortlessly adjusts.

The aesthetic rules of the sacred Japanese gardens on the Kyushu island have crossed the ages and continents to feed a westernised version with the Zen gardens - we imported the idea we had of them without respecting their religious, poetic, cultural and philosophical symbolism. But the main idea has remained - that of a place of purification, where the spirit finds a state of grace in balance with the forces of the Universe. Mastery of this subtle, codified arrangement and knowledge of the practices associated with it reflect a person's level of education and are a lifelong journey, a culmination as much as a road to follow.

1.5. Mediaeval Gardens

From the Middle Ages onwards, vegetable gardens and orchards enabled Parisian hospices to make substantial savings, but also to occupy people who were prone to vagrancy and begging. These hospital gardens were developed in the 17th century to occupy the "mad and insane" in the hospices and asylums [151]. These gardens of the Middle Ages have been revived and idealised in modern times. They have become an expression of nostalgia for a vanished paradise, a time when religious communities organised a perfect world far from the suffering and turpitude of the world. Yet the sacredness of mediaeval gardens is real - their architectural logic and creative visualisation were inspired by a representation of the divine. Their design was guided by codes, rules and specifications that combined religious symbolism with the need to satisfy everyday requirements (food, clothing, care).

It is worth remembering that there was a very strong interaction between garden design and the Catholic Church during this period. Mediaeval gardens [152] and the artistic representations associated with them were tools for spreading the Christian faith. The Middle Ages were a time when the Catholic Church was establishing its authority and its dogma, notably through 14 of the 21 ecumenical councils organised in its history. At the time when cathedrals were being built, gardens were the vehicle for an ideal representation of the greatness of Christianity, as described by the Fathers of the Church and inspiring a divine vision. These gardens fed the imagination and helped to construct an ideal vision of the world, combining the four elements (earth, air, fire, water) in a square, in a circle evoking the vault of heaven. They are very often organised in the form of a symbolic cross, with a fountain or tree of life as its centre of gravity. The garden's universal appeal can be seen both in the reality of the monasteries and in their depictions in paintings and tapestries. The presence of collections of medicinal plants grown in squares surrounded by boxwood - the Herbularium - provided the monks with plants such as thyme, sage, rosemary, mint, lavender and oregano, whose preparations were used to soothe the sick.

The *Book of Simple Medicines* by Platearius [153], an eminent 12th-century botanist from the Salerno School of Medicine (Schola Salernita), was a key reference. In it, he described four hundred and ninety-seven medicinal plants and how to prepare them to make remedies for the illnesses of his time. This work complements the *Physica* [154] by von Bingen (1098-1170), a Benedictine abbess who knew how to observe nature and heal with plants. The therapy used in this medicinal garden was therefore the work of the herbalist, who acted as both apothecary and physician. His empirical knowledge of plants guided him in the preparation of decoctions, infusions, macerations, broths, powdered plants, poultices... the symbolic images went beyond the power of plants. In this way, *the Song of Songs* was used as a starting point for a threaded metaphor. The care provided by the herbalist through the use of medicinal plants is a subtle blend of real therapy and divine allegory. This practice of healing with plants is currently known as phytotherapy and is distinct from the healing that can be attributed to the garden. Does the garden really heal and/or is it simply the messenger of the Church? And to put the question further, what are we referring to when we say that this medicinal garden heals? The Church has given each plant a symbolic message:

- The lily's whiteness symbolised purity and the Immaculate Conception.
- The columbine, with its five petals, was compared to five doves, and the dove to the Holy Spirit.
- The iris, with its three petals, suggested the Holy Trinity
- The strawberry plant, hidden among the grasses, symbolised humility; its white flower, purity; its three-lobed leaf, the Trinity; its red fruit, the Passion.

1.6. Andalusian Gardens

Unlike the mediaeval garden, which has not survived the test of time and of which we only see contemporary versions inspired by the Middle Ages, you can still visit the gardens of the Alhambra in Granada, the Alcazar in Seville or Cordoba in Andalusia.

The religious dimension regularly amplifies the power of the imagination in contemplating reality. This begins, of course, with the mastery of water, which in arid or even desert territories always takes on the value of a superhuman feat - both in terms of the scale of the work involved and the techniques and inventiveness required.

Their blend of inspiration from ancient, mediaeval and Muslim culture has produced jewels whose magnificence ranges from abundance to luxuriance to harmony. It's a challenge made all the more impressive by the fact that it is played out in the most arid of territories, where mastery of water is the key to the flowering of life. Beyond the demonstration of power and the attempt to produce an earthly representation of the Mohammedan paradise, the Hispano-Moorish gardens of Granada and Seville were a regular source of inspiration for the perfect expression of the five senses. An atmosphere of sensuality prefigures a paradisiacal vision where all desires are satisfied and sensuality flourishes in an intimate relationship where man has mastered nature.

1.7. English Gardens

The passion and talents of the English for gardening are indisputable. In Great Britain, you can visit magical places where a genius for spatial planning, a mastery of plants and a talent for making the hand of man disappear behind nature are superimposed, giving the illusion that these jewels, which require constant supervision, have developed spontaneously around the manor houses and residences that they accompany. The same is true of English lawns, which are a benchmark of excellence in the world. Originally, the aim was to demonstrate political and economic power by occupying a territory and using manpower to maintain a perfect lawn by hand, with no other intention than to decorate. A recent publication set out the health benefits of an English lawn [155].

2. Sanatoria

Before going any further, it is worth pausing for a moment to consider the history of sanatoria, which in themselves represent an interesting illustration of the influence of the cultural heritage of gardens on public health policies [41]. Sanatoria disappeared from the French institutional and health landscape over forty years ago. Although their name is still associated with tuberculosis, today it evokes only a distant therapeutic past, where notions of "fresh air," "*climatic cure*" and "*hygienism*" are blurred together.

As cultural objects, sanatoria embody the investment of an entire generation - particularly of doctors - in the fight against tuberculosis, of which few traces remain beyond the buildings themselves. But their architecture remains mute today: like an instrument that has become foreign for lack of regular use, the sanatorium can only be understood if we know its ins and outs, particularly its medical and architectural aspects. From the mid-19th century onwards, sanatoria played an essential role in Europe, combining architecture and medical devices in a single concept.

Sanatoriums as a means of studying the relationship between the environment and health are all the more interesting since, after their closure at the end of the Second World War, a good number of them were converted into nursing homes.

The claim of "modernity" which the partisans of the sanatorium - doctors as well as architects - never ceased to declare is an ideological construct which does not stand up well to the historical analysis of its foundations. The sanatorium is a sanitary type resulting from the medical thought of the beginning of the 19th century and which continued until the 1960s when we saw the last traces of it disappear. It is particularly surprising and paradoxical that sanatorium methods were thus able to impose themselves on the medical world: this medical world was mainly guided by a demand to respect a scientific logic based on empiricism. It was above all a question of putting sick people in the best conditions to fight against disease. For decades, the medical world had adopted a logic that went against the current of scientific progress. The progress initiated by the work of Laennec, Villemin and Koch gave doctors new weapons to act directly on infectious agents.

However, sanatorium architecture was able to impose itself throughout Europe for almost a century - particularly in France, Germany and Switzerland - to the point of becoming an essential institution in medical practices and is the setting in which Thomas Mann built a myth with his novel "*Der Zauberberg*" (The Magic Mountain).

Tuberculosis has many symptoms, usually discreet, which used to make its diagnosis more difficult at an early stage. The main manifestations were fever and sweats. The clinical picture could evolve towards general weight loss, sometimes combined with anorexia and digestive disorders. Asthenia - irrepressible physical and intellectual weariness - was also considered a predictive marker of the disease. These symptoms were generally variable according to the patients. Some functional signs indicated lung disease in particular. First there was the coughing, an "essential, cardinal, constant sign." Rather dry and early in the morning, it was accompanied by sputum as the disease progressed. These expectorations formed mucous sputum containing the purulent matter evacuated by the tubercles into the bronchi. Accompanied by blood, this sputum was the sign of hemoptysis, linked to lesions of the trachea, bronchi or lung tissue. It was a classic manifestation of pulmonary tuberculosis although it was not specific to this disease. General fatigue and chest pain were often added to these symptoms.

Adding to the physical examination by the doctor, from the end of the 19th century onwards, the field of radiography revolutionised the diagnosis of tuberculosis by making it possible to have a precise image of the lungs. According to the state of evolution of the disease, the patient was directed or not towards various health establishments - largely depending on how contagious the person was.

Tuberculosis was not only a serious disease, difficult to cure, but it also led to a social downgrading of the sick. Before social insurance came to their aid, working class people who were sick with tuberculosis were invariably drawn into a downward spiral of social precariousness and worsening health, the only foreseeable outcome of which was death.

At the beginning of the 20th century, an English study established a significant relationship between the size of housing and the probability of its inhabitants developing tuberculosis.

At the end of the nineteenth and beginning of the twentieth centuries, tuberculosis sanatoria developed the therapeutic role of the garden, described by Grandvoinnet, in the notion of "sublime isolation in nature." The architecture of sanatoria suggests the notion of an ecological approach to illness. Grandvoinnet gives the example of "*the tuberculosis pavilions at the Boucicaut hospital in Paris (1898), where the best exposed gable ended in a fully glazed winter garden accessible from the patient's' ward.*" The decree of 1920 August 10th stipulated that "*every sanatorium must be surrounded by a park reserved for it or have a wood nearby for the organization of the training cure.*" No studies have confirmed the benefits of these gardens in the treatment of tuberculosis. The sanatoriums disappeared with the discovery of streptomycin in 1946, leaving many buildings empty, some of which were later converted into nursing homes or hospitals.

However, as a legacy of these decades of architectural therapeutic practices, there are thousands of pages of theses and reports describing the hypotheses put forward by doctors and architects which were then deconstructed by the poor effectiveness or ineffectiveness of the solutions recommended. The sanatorium project was thus a perpetual "bricolage," like the incessant renewal of a toolbox made up of disparate elements. Doctors and architects drew from it, the elements needed to design a sanatorium as a technical instrument, based on apparent scientific rigor. Consequently, when sanatoriums were disaffected, their conversion was a real headache for institutions, as there was no real classification to characterise their design.

3. The Concept of "Therapeutic Garden" or "Healing Garden"

The term "therapeutic garden" emerged in the 1990s, without the benefit of a precise conceptual framework. It was a translation of the term "healing garden," which suggests the healing capacity of the garden. There is no single name for these gardens: care garden, sensory garden, garden of the senses, therapeutic garden or garden with a therapeutic vocation. The variety of names used sums up the imprecision of the concept. For the remainder of our exploration, we will use the term "therapeutic garden" to designate this set of concepts. Therapeutic gardens are rooted in the history of gardens. We have described the extent to which gardens, through their representation of an ideal form of nature, suggests that gardens are rooted in health benefits.

One of the first publications to establish the role of therapeutic gardens was the work of Ulrich (1984) [156], who observed that the view of a wooded park from the window of a hospital room accelerated convalescence after a cholecystectomy. Ulrich noted that the group of 23 patients with a view of trees had a significantly shorter average length of hospitalisation than the group of 23 patients with a view of a wall (7.96 days and 8.70 days respectively).

This study, conducted in a Pennsylvania hospital between 1972 and 1981, excluded patients under 20 and over 69. Forty years on, this study is regularly cited as a demonstration of the benefits of gardens on the health of hospital patients.

However, we have some difficulty in considering that Ulrich's study can be considered a definitive demonstration and proof of the beneficial effect of gardens on health. On the one hand, because the connection between the garden and the participants in the study does not establish any direct relationship, and on the other because the result measured is not, strictly speaking, an inflection on a health marker, but more precisely a reduction in convalescence time.

If it was so easy to demonstrate, it's surprising that in over forty years it hasn't been possible to produce more convincing evidence. And if this is not the case, it should be done as a matter of urgency. Yet even today, most popular articles on 'therapeutic gardens' are introduced by a phrase such as "since Ulrich's work in 1984, it is no longer necessary to demonstrate the beneficial effects of gardens on health..."

Professor and landscape architect Cooper Marcus [157] has defined the therapeutic garden as follows: "*A general term for gardens that have a positive effect on stress and other positive influences on patients.*" The image and representation of the garden ideal designates it as a space suitable for a therapeutic purpose. The social construct has made it a benevolent and popular place, and its development is subject to fewer financial and regulatory constraints than buildings. For example, Ulrich [73] points out the difference between the USD $1.8 billion budgeted for the renovation of the hospital in Houston, Texas and the very modest cost of creating therapeutic gardens.

The arguments in favour of therapeutic gardens overlap, some drawing on nature, others on age-old practices, and still others on the growing attraction of urban populations for close contact with plants. Each of them is likely to be convincing, without necessarily having a solid scientific basis.

A large proportion of the articles currently published, both scientific and popular, support the idea that the health benefits of gardens are an established notion that no longer needs to be demonstrated.

A literature review carried out by Howarth, Brettle and Hardman [158] in 2017 presents a recent version of this. In this scoping review of publications from the last 25 years, Howarth analysed a selection of 67 articles. The conclusions of this literature review identify the beneficial effects of therapeutic gardens in reducing obesity and depression and improving social ties, physical activity and appetite. In the discussion, however, the author expresses a major reservation about the methodological rigor and lack of robustness of the protocols used. This is one of the main limitations highlighted by Howarth, who state: *"There is a significant lack of studies that have used robust experimental approaches."* There is a paradox between the proposed conclusion that therapeutic gardens are beneficial to health and the methodological fragility of the studies.

One might wonder whether the gardens laid out in geriatric institutions are not simply a return to a 'normal' environment for residents, compared with interior architecture that often resembles an impoverished environment.

Before talking about 'therapeutic gardens', should we not consider certain forms of architectural abuse? Souchon, Nogues and Jibidar [159] described architectural ill-treatment as a set of architectural shortcomings or failings linked to inadequate artificial lighting, the absence of air conditioning, poor building aesthetics, poor acoustic quality, unsuitable flooring, a lack of privacy, and excessive or inadequate security. The presence of a garden in a nursing home or hospital could be likened to an "oxygen bubble" or an island of good treatment, made available to patients/residents to compensate for an unstimulating or even "impoverished" environment in medico-social institutions.

Societal expectations about gardens take precedence over the need for scientific validation. If therapeutic gardens do not have evidence-based benefits, then enthusiasm to support them runs the risk of waning as people debate the budgetary constraints that are constantly being exerted on institutions. Scientific validation and proofs would provide benchmarks for healthcare professionals so that they can usefully promote and guide the use of gardens.

The knowledge acquired about the relationship between the garden and the residents in a geriatric institution could contribute to better design and use of the physical environment for the older adults.

We need an appropriate context to translate the knowledge that we have acquired so far about environmental enrichment to human models. Gardens are a good place to do this. They are not subject to the stringent regulatory standards that apply to all areas within a geriatric institution, and the cost of fitting out garden spaces for experimental work is not too high. As we have just seen, however, gardens benefit from a significant bias stemming from the social constructs around them. Their status as a representation of a form of human ideal gives them an aura that is often difficult to challenge. In the context of this research on the transposition of the principles of environmental enrichment for the older adults, it was necessary to establish demanding methodological rules so as not to reproduce the difficulties encountered by previous studies on the physical environment in institutions.

4. The Enriched Garden Concept

Transposing the principles of environmental enrichment to humans required the use of a space which would enable studies to be performed using a robust methodology. The choice of a garden space quickly became obvious because it met all the essential criteria for conducting this research.

Combining a garden with an enriched environment offers the possibility of combining the respective advantages of both in the same space, forming an innovative concept: an enriched garden. An innovative concept must satisfy several major requirements to ensure its validity and longevity. The concept was described and theorised in Ogden and Richards' book "*The meaning of meaning: A study of the influence of language upon thought and of the science of symbolism*" published in 1923 [160].

Ogden and Richards' approach was originally designed to explain and remedy misunderstandings between expressed and perceived thought (Figure

12). Wilson went into more detail on the need to define a conceptual dimension in his book *"Thinking with concepts"*[161]. He establishes patterns of thought on three different levels: the facts, their value(s) and the concept(s) they evoke. This distinction between 'facts', the primary level of designation of an object of interest, and the higher level of 'concept' suggests that beyond semantics, the meaning of words has a scope that engages notions and values that go beyond their objective value. It is in this sense that Wilson suggests that when an expression has a conceptual dimension, it should be isolated in order to analyse and understand it as a concept, and to describe its attributes and associated extensions. Drawing inspiration from Wilson and Wittgenstein [162], who had worked on the philosophy of language, Gerring [163] established and published a framework in 1999 for validating the formation of a concept. Beyond words, concepts are intended to build theories, and without a well-defined framework, neither concept nor theory is possible. As Kaplan wrote in 1965 [164]: *"the proper concepts are needed to formulate a good theory, but we need a good theory to arrive at the proper concept."*

Gerring emphasises that research must be based on these fundamental prerequisites, because his continuous exploratory work has regularly led him to define innovative concepts whose durability and relevance are at risk of being rendered invalid by use and time.

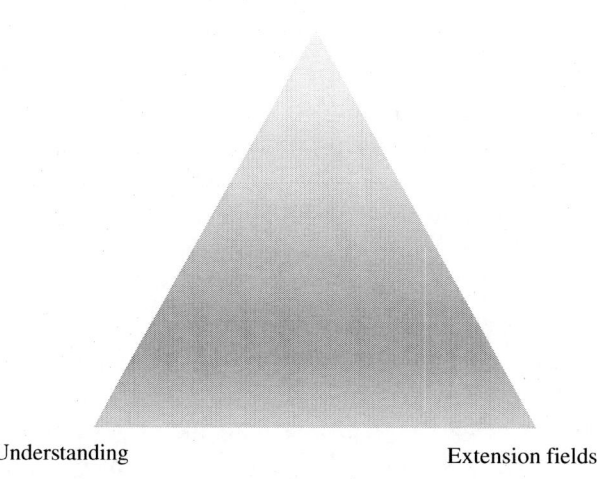

Figure 12. Simplified representation of the concept established by Ogden & Richards (1923).

If we have gone through the process of defining a precise concept, it is because our research work requires the chosen research environment to have a precise definition. This environmental concept had to free itself from social constructs and, in the particular case of gardens, from their historical, philosophical, cultural and political heritage. In reality, this was only a transitional phase in the development of the ideal environment resulting from the transposition of laboratory work to the human environment.

4.1. Designation

There are three strategies for choosing the name of a concept:

1. Use a word from current vocabulary and give it a conceptual framework
2. Invent a word - usually from Greek or Latin roots
3. Combine 2 or more words to combine their respective meanings.

In the specific context of the "enriched garden," the third strategy has been chosen:

- The first word, "garden," appeals to a universally accepted dimension, but has very different meanings in different cultures and civilizations. It offers a general framework; however, whose etymology refers to an enclosed space - in the Germanic language the word "gart" means fence - which in Latin formed "hortus gardinus." The term "garden" can be translated into many languages without changing its meaning.
- The second term, "enriched," is directly inherited from the concept described in the work initiated by Hebb and continued over the last few decades on enriched environments - with its two associated dimensions: enrichment of the environment and scientific research.

The term 'enriched garden' is a combination of enriched environment and garden space.

By combining the two, 'enriched garden' suggests a garden which, through its enrichment - in a version adapted from the enrichment achieved by Hebb on the animal model - is a beneficial space for health, and a scientific device for pursuing research activities.

The translation of 'enriched garden' is:

- French: jardin enrichi
- German: bereicherter garten
- In Italian: giardino arricchito
- In Chinese: 丰富的花园 (fēng fù de huā yuán) using the Chinese characters used to designate "enriched environment" in Chinese literature.

4.2. Understanding

In "*What makes a concept good? A critical framework for understanding concept formation in social sciences*" Gerring asserted that it was not possible to impose a universal understanding of a concept through naming alone. Following in the footsteps of Ogden and Richards, Gerring recommended characterizing the concept by a list of eight criteria that form its general architecture and ensure its shared understanding - whereas the definitions proposed by dictionaries would risk opening the field to interpretations. These interpretations are potentially latent insofar as the garden, as described above, carries a strong dimension of subjectivity - linked to its social construct.

The concept of the "enriched garden" is relevant and coherent in terms of Gerring's eight criteria.

The eight criteria for developing a concept are as follows:

- Familiarity:
  Would the concept be familiar when presented to an academic audience?
  Understanding is instantaneous as soon as the term is perceived by an audience familiar with the concept of an enriched environment. The difficulty in understanding this term lies mainly in appreciating the type of enrichment contained.
- Resonance:
  Does the chosen name immediately ring a bell?
  The presence of the word "garden" in the name creates a high degree of familiarity, which can lead to the concept of an "enriched garden" being perceived as less familiar than a "conventional garden."
- Parsimony:

Is it possible to describe it soberly?
The simplicity of the terms used is a factor favouring adoption of the concept. The characterization of the main attributes associated with it: frequentation, appropriation and health benefits reinforce its legitimacy while imposing requirements.
- Consistency:
Is there an immediately perceptible logic between the name and the attributes?
This concept associates gardens and enriched environments, which ensures the consistency of its attributes and objectives.
- Differentiation:
Can the associated concept be clearly differentiated from closely related concepts? Is it operational and clear?
Differentiation is formed by its three major attributes (enrichment, scientific research activity and appropriation)
- Depth:
Are there many properties that institutions will associate with this concept?
The principle of scientific research that underpins the concept and the health objectives that accompany this concept form its depth.
- Theoretical utility:
Does the concept make a useful contribution to its field of action?
The concept opens up a new field in the development and use of gardens compared with current perceptions. Although this perception is sometimes polluted by the received idea that any garden, with no specific attributes, can offer the same functions as any other garden, the concept of the enriched garden offers new possibilities.
- Semantic field utility:
Will institutions find this new concept really useful?
The concept of the enriched garden opens up a wide range of possibilities (see extensions).

There is a difficulty on the criterion of "resonance" in spontaneously perceiving the additional contribution of the "enriched garden" to the "garden"; all the more so as the garden, in the minds of most people, naturally has a positive effect on health, all the more so in the context of the contemporary quest for nature. The closest concept - that of the healing garden - although it does not have a well-established conceptual framework, competes semantically with the "enriched garden."

4.3. The Attributes of the Enriched Garden

The value of a concept is measured by the relevance and interest of its attributes. We have identified three essential attributes associated with the enriched garden.

4.3.1. Ownership
Ownership is an essential issue when the environment is considered to be a determining factor in the resident's quality of life and health. There are few publications looking at the process of appropriation of the environment by a resident in nursing homes. Our research involves identifying the different stages in the process of residents taking ownership of the enriched garden and characterizing the modes of ownership through their interactions with the garden.

4.3.2. The Associated Scientific Approach
Inspired by the concept of an enriched environment, the enriched garden is, in its intention and design, a tool supported by a scientific methodology. As we saw in the chapter *"the physical environment in geriatric institutions,"* one of the difficulties in identifying the effect of the environment on health lies in the fragility of the protocols used for observational or interventional studies. This scientific approach, based on existing knowledge about environmental enrichment, is designed to identify and analyse the potential benefits of enriched gardens on human health. It does not consider these health benefits as a given, but as an essential parameter to be assessed scientifically.

4.3.3. Modularity of Health and Well-Being Benefits by Adjusting the Enrichment of the Garden
The enrichment of the garden is a fundamental element of the enriched garden concept. It is based on the design of specific modules that will guide visitors through the garden towards interactions and stimuli that target identified problems and weaknesses: cognitive, behavioural and mood problems, functional independence, walking and balance. These modules need to be designed with relevance in mind, and their benefits need to be evaluated within the framework of appropriate protocols.

The modules used in an enriched garden also need to be chosen with the right modularity for the population using the garden.

4.4. Extensions of the Enriched Garden

Ogden and Richards in 1923 and then Gerring in 1999, emphasised the need for extensions to be associated with a concept if it is to be established. A concept can only really be a concept if it has wider dimensions than the simple domain in which it was conceived. These extensions constitute an empirical opening towards other fields of application. Some of these extensions are observable when the concept is formulated, others not yet; but they are part of the field of possibilities to which these extensions can make an ephemeral, evolving or lasting contribution - a notion described by Depeyre (165) in an article entitled: *"Dynamic capabilities: problems of defining and operationalizing the concept."*

One of the restrictions experienced by the notion of the therapeutic garden is its limited application to the specific field of medico-social institutions. The definitions given by the authors of therapeutic gardens are based on two concepts: the health benefits of the garden and its location within a medico-social institution. This notion, linked to a specific place (the institution), does not facilitate extensions to other uses. The "enriched garden" provides greater flexibility for considering ways to extend its use. Transposing the concept of an enriched environment to the garden facilitates extensions to other uses.

This notion of extensions associated with the enriched garden is developed more fully in the last chapter of this work" *Enriched environments: Extensions and perspectives."* It indicates vertical and horizontal dimensions based on the modularity of enrichment, which enables each garden to be adapted to the health issues of the population concerned.

This analysis of the concept of an enriched garden, based on the Ogden and Richards triangle, assumes that the concept is dynamic. Depending on the empirical demonstrations of future extensions, it is possible to observe a conceptual stretching - in which the fields of what is possible but also impossible are described more broadly. A fundamental question underlying the statement of criteria for understanding the enriched garden is that of the "organization" to which this concept is addressed. Wittgenstein offers a warning on this point, pointing out that the rigor imposed in defining a concept constitutes an error by failing to measure the richness and diversity of possible extensions: *"We tend to think that there must, for example, be something common to all games, and that this common property justifies our applying the general term 'game' to all games; whereas in fact games form a family whose members have family resemblances. Some of them have the same nose, others the same eyebrows, and still others the same gait; and these resemblances overlap. The idea that a general concept is a property common to its particular cases is linked to other primitive and overly simple ideas about the structure of language."*

The same is true if we consider comparing the experiments carried out in enriched gardens created in private homes with those in urban spaces. There is also an important dimension attached to this notion of extensions, concerning the crossing of cultural boundaries. As we saw above, environmental enrichment has been adopted by the international scientific community, and research work has been carried out in laboratories all over the world. What about the concept of enriched gardens?

5. Enriched Gardens - Operational Dimensions

5.1. Enriched Gardens: A Permanent Invitation

The principle underlying the design of an enriched garden is to centre the technical and architectural choices around the vulnerabilities and problems encountered by the people who will use it. The usual approach to landscape design for a traditional garden is based on an analysis of the environment in which the garden is to be located. This environmental analysis is used to assess the constraints and opportunities for development, depending on the spatial orientation, the nature of the soil, the ecosystem and the climate. When designing an enriched garden, the first step is to identify the general profile of future users and then to carry out an environmental assessment. The challenge associated with this approach is to design a space that is adapted to the users, and that minimises their apprehension about using it.

The fundamental approach to designing an enriched environment for older adults living in geriatric institutions is to place the individual (the resident) at the heart of the issues. The principle of enriching the garden was inspired by the approach adopted by research into enriched environments. It has been adapted to take account of the specific features of life in a nursing home and life with Alzheimer's disease. We designed the enrichment elements based on a multidisciplinary constructivist approach involving healthcare professionals, carers, landscapers and craftsmen. Each enrichment module was designed with the same working group, around specific questions such as:

- How can the spatial orientation of a resident with Alzheimer's disease be improved?

- What environment could minimise anxiety disorders?

The challenge associated with this approach is to design a space that is adapted to the users, and that minimises any reservations they have about using it. Cohen-Mansfield's survey [118] of 320 nursing homes in the United States shows that 62% of residents make little or no use of the garden - a low level of use explained either by weather conditions, by the distance from the buildings being too great, or by accessibility issues (doors too heavy or difficult to operate). This low level of use was also observed in the many nursing homes we visited in France.

Participatory working groups involving residents, family carers and healthcare professionals worked intensively over several months to transform this highly conceptual approach about how to transpose the enriched environment into detailed technical design elements. The main obstacles to use of the garden identified during these consultations were as follows:

- The garden is too far away or not visible from inside the buildings, reducing the visual appeal to residents.
- Weather conditions: too cold, too hot, rainy, too bright, or windy. The contrast between a controlled atmosphere inside the establishments and a more or less favourable atmosphere outside can make residents nervous about going outside. This apprehension is reinforced by the level of frailty of the residents.
- The architecture of the garden is such that you can see all of it without entering. As a result, the garden has the status of a landscape garden that can be viewed from a distance, without any perceived interest in "venturing out."
- The absence or lack of rest areas (benches, handrails) and stable surfaces for walking often discourages residents from going there unaccompanied.
- Evergreen vegetation that changes little or not at all with the seasons does not inspire the sense of discovery that a variety of plants would offer, with flowers and foliage whose colours change a little every day.
- White or too-light flooring that reflects the sun's rays and creates visual glare is a further nuisance. Similarly, too steep a slope or the presence of steps discourage regular visits.

It became apparent that the garden, while a space much appreciated by residents and their carers, had to meet a large number of requirements. These requirements are all the more important to understand as there are currently very few technical and regulatory standards governing the layout of a nursing home garden. Every detail is likely to create an obstacle to the use of the garden and negate the desire to visit it. The collaborative working groups that we conducted with healthcare professionals, residents and family carers led us to formulate a set of specifications for a garden that we have entitled "the permanent invitation," following the models described by Grahn and Bengtsson.

The suggestions made by the participants were formulated as a group, giving priority to meeting the needs of the residents, while integrating the technical constraints set out by the technicians and the landscape dimension emphasised by the landscape designers. The participants' contributions were collected and analysed collectively, identifying each person's expertise:

- *Health professionals:* doctors, nurses, occupational therapists, psychomotor therapists, psychologists, recreational therapists, and art therapists. Their contribution involved assessing the residents' abilities to interact intuitively with these modules.
- *Relatives and residents:* They were recruited from among volunteers involved in the life of their establishment. Residents with an interest in gardens and with the cognitive capacity to take an active part in the workshops were also invited (early stage Alzheimer's disease).
- *Craftsmen and industrial manufacturers:* the aim of their participation in these workshops was to ensure that they had a precise understanding of the challenges and objectives of the enrichment modules for use by residents, so that they could provide the most appropriate technical solutions.
- *The landscape architects:* Their task was to adapt the modules to optimise their integration into the landscape, so that these modules appeared in the garden as if they had grown with the plants.

As a result of this design process using iterative steps, the "enriched garden" is a new environment to be conquered. The issues at stake are: 1) the validation of its effects on the health of the older adults, 2) the use and sense of ownership that it will provide residents and, most importantly, 3) the information that it will provide with a view to extending its concept to all the shared spaces of geriatric institutions. It is therefore from these different perspectives that we have transcribed our reading of the design and evaluation of the main dimensions of an enriched garden.

- What kind of architecture and design help to ensure that residents in institutions use their space regularly and make it their own?
- How do enriched gardens contribute to the health and quality of life of the older adults?
- What lessons can we learn from these studies about extending this concept to all shared spaces in nursing homes?

5.1.1. What Kind of Architecture and Design Help to Ensure That Residents in Institutions Use Their Space Regularly and Make It Their Own?

The primary challenge of this enriched space is not that it exists and offers positive effects on the health of residents, but primarily that it is frequented and adopted by residents.

This notion of appropriation is all the more relevant as it is supported by numerous works in the literature, in particular by researchers in the social sciences and political science, geographers and urban planners who study the notion of territory, territoriality, heritage and public space (in relation to identity and collective memory).

We need to define and understand what is meant by "appropriate space" and by or for whom. The notion of appropriation seems to be common knowledge in the social sciences, as if its definition were self-evident. Yet it brings together a number of very different domains, each of which requires its own special understanding.

5.2. Spatial Appropriation and Health

The sense of spatial appropriation, and in particular the feeling of being at home in a defined place, plays a key role in the development of social identity, especially for the older adults, as a vital element in the perception of their own identity. In 1991, Ringel [166] described the notion of spatial appropriation as being directly associated with quality of life and mental health.

And yet, although spatial appropriation is essential, it is described relatively little or poorly in the literature, especially when it comes to a major change of residence such as when an older adult enters a nursing home.

Geographers, sociologists and urban planners have carried out a significant number of studies on the appropriation of public space by citizens. They distinguish several significant, even different, levels of ownership:

- the first meaning generally associated with this notion is the legal and economic dimension, which places the relationship with the environment in a patrimonial value - property then represents a key element in terms of resources and social status. This legal and economic relationship to the environment is determined by values such as public/private, accessible/reserved, free/charged, for sale/rent, etc.).

We quickly discover that appropriation can express more relationships to a space other than simple private ownership. It remains to be seen how these other forms of appropriation can be defined. This needs to be described in particular in relation to the notion of use:

- exclusive use: established within a framework of competing for limited goods. This exclusivity can be individual, but is more often collective, based on concrete but restricted groups (such as the family) or broader social categories (such as gender). It can arise from strictly material or functional reasons, but also from more directly social ones: appropriation is then synonymous with enclosure through various material devices.
- autonomous use, corresponding to the fact of using space freely, or at least without any explicit social constraints.
- Control of space is a third meaning and should not be underestimated. Here, control is often exercised by intermediaries, who are not necessarily autonomous in their relationship with the space. Rather, it's a question of power, of domination, exercised by apparatuses or institutions, such as a state over its territory.

These forms of appropriation are inseparable from intentions, perceptions and representations, and even imaginary or ideological constructs. Other orders of meaning are more clearly part of this ideological register. This is the case of learning and familiarization, conceived as cognitive internalization: appropriating a space here means acquiring theoretical and practical knowledge, know-how and skills that enable you to move around it without getting lost, but also to use it in a relevant or strategic way.

Affective attachment or, even more profoundly, what we might call "existential" appropriation, is another aspect to consider. This is the feeling of belonging, of being at home somewhere. This sense of appropriation is then transformed into a feeling of belonging. The relationship with places is experienced as reciprocal: a place is ours because we belong to it, and it is part of us because we are part of it.

Finally, to these relatively common meanings we propose to add "symbolic" or "identity-based" appropriation: a portion of land space (a place or a set of places) is associated with a social group or category to the point of becoming one of its attributes, i.e., helping to define its social identity. This is how we commonly speak of middle-class neighbourhoods and working-class suburbs, but categorization can also be based on nationality, religion, political leanings, age, gender and so on. The symbolic appropriation of space can be made through signage, commemorative monuments, church buildings etc.

The inequalities are perhaps even greater, though sometimes less visible, if we understand appropriation to mean mastery of one's own living space, i.e., autonomy of use. In contrast to those who use their own space as they see fit - a space they have produced or had produced in their own image and to their own measure - there are those who can only make do with spaces produced for them, according to the image others have of their needs, their criteria, their very value one might say. Appropriation is opposite to both assignment and expropriation (or expulsion).

Thus, over the course of a lifetime, a relationship to space and the environment is established that is strongly conditioned by these different forms of social constructs, as well as by individual experience. A person who has never owned their own home, or who has been evicted from it, or a person who has never been part of a social group, will no doubt develop very different relationships with the environment in which they live.

This relationship with space, and a person's ability to appropriate it, is a particularly rich subject when associated with the issue of ageing. When dependency makes it more difficult to move around, the space available for appropriation shrinks. Older people have to give up certain spaces that have become progressively less accessible, or even completely inaccessible.

Similarly, for those who remain lucid, the central question about losing ownership of space that inevitably arises in old age is: what to choose? To stay or to leave? Should a person abandon, at the right moment, their home, their ecological niche, and slip into an often-unstimulating collective universe that drowns identities in a confused indifference? What are we to think about the conditions that enable a process of de-appropriation, leading to a re-appropriation of an undoubtedly different nature? This initial reflection on a theme that will become increasingly important illustrates a third application of the environmental perspective. This is the introduction of the temporal dimension, by examining how the evolution of life cycles modifies people's relationship to space.

We thus construct a relationship with the space in which we live that is based not only on the material or patrimonial dimension, but also, and perhaps above all, on an idealised relationship with ourselves. In order to claim ownership of a given space, without being able to produce a certificate of ownership, the individual produces signs which are an act of spatial marking that can take different expressions. This may take the form of fencing off an occupied space, planting a tree, grazing animals, street demonstrations, graffiti on walls, statues, linguistic signs or, more simply, a piece of clothing on the back of a chair. These claims are sometimes inspired by a desire to denounce social inequalities - equivalent to asking "*why is it that the place I live and occupy is collectively owned and not mine*?"

From a more qualitative angle, this spatial claim also sometimes concerns the living environment, whether it's a place of work, leisure, study, religious or political practice, care or convalescence. It can be a setting that is more or less valued for its aesthetics, functionality and prestige.

This framework, while asserted, can be identified by its shortcomings (lack of facilities, unsuitability, etc.) or by its harmful effects (pollution) or even by the form of stigmatization it imposes.

On all these points, we can observe an undeniably strong hierarchy [167-168]. At one end of the social scale, a minority selects, accumulates, occupies and fully enjoys vast quantities of space, in almost all respects this space is considered to be of "better quality," well positioned, or at any rate of great value because it is highly valued. For example, the Pinçon-Charlot couple's research focuses primarily on the "*great fortunes*" of the wealthy, but also on certain leaders, elected and/or senior civil servants, and even local notables, who benefit from prestigious buildings and other elements of public heritage while in office. At the other end of the scale, we find the minority made up of those who find themselves on the street, but also the majority of the so-called "working" and even "middle" classes who invest a large part of their budget in their main home, and who are often forced to choose between the depreciated housing estates on the outskirts of town, or a home that is certainly central, but also more cramped and more expensive. As for home ownership, for many it remains a forbidden adventure, or one that is all the more risky and restrictive because of their limited resources and can even turn into a new form of "alienation."

Thus, our questioning of spatial appropriation as a vector of the relationship that an individual establishes with his or her environment carries essential information not only on the methodology that enables us to apprehend it, but also on the social, cultural and ideological constructs that we associate with our living spaces.

These notions feed into a "holistic rhetoric," an ideological discourse on the "collective" and the "common notions" that conceal the social inequalities, conflicts of interest and power relations that permeate human communities.

These considerations are essential for establishing the framework and modalities of the relationship between an individual and their environment. They were a fundamental prerequisite in the planning and design of the "enriched garden" concept. Indeed, these interactions will profoundly determine the salutogenic vision to which the environment can contribute as part of an approach to health and well-being in institutions, but also in the various living situations where environmental enrichment could be implemented. The "enriched garden" is an experimental facility that supports this transfer of laboratory work with mice to the human setting. It was therefore essential to develop a rigorous approach to define its characterization in the human environment, and all the more so that of frail people such as the residents of geriatric institutions.

For these interactions to take place, and for the older adults to benefit from them, it is important that they are willing and encouraged to visit the enriched garden spontaneously and regularly. To this end, a series of measures have been identified and implemented to meet the main challenges of this frequent usage.

In terms of frequency, we have adopted the principles used in laboratory studies of enriched environments, i.e., an average of 4 to 5 exhibitions per week, each lasting 15 to 30 minutes. At this stage, this frequency is only a working hypothesis, to be refined in the future by comparative studies on the effectiveness (or otherwise) of varying this rhythm on health markers.

It is clear, however, that in the context of nursing home life, such attendance can only be the result of a voluntary approach by the resident. That is why we have described the main elements involved in voluntary attendance.

The principle behind the design of an enriched garden is to focus technical and architectural choices on the fragilities and problems encountered by the people who will be using it. The usual approach to landscape design for a conventional garden is based on an analysis of the environment in which the garden is to be planted. This environmental analysis enables us to qualify the constraints and opportunities for development, according to spatial orientation, soil type, ecosystem and climate. When designing an enriched garden, the first step is to identify the general profile of future users, and then to carry out an environmental assessment. This progressive rise in the demand for attention in the environment, which Grahn and Bengtsson have called the challenge gradient, is an important aspect of health promotion in the overall design of the health garden and reflects the healing process. The garden must therefore offer a continuum of environmental qualities, from passive experience of nature to active interaction with people and natural elements.

Inspiring design aims to meet the need for access to nature by offering variation and change in daily life, freedom to choose from alternatives, and stimulation of the senses and intellect, and is therefore consistent with salutogenic strategies that support salutary factors. Comfortable design must be considered in the environment as a whole, so that everyone, whatever their physical and cognitive condition, can use and experience the garden in its entirety.

Each specific target group, and indeed each individual, has a wide range of preferences and needs during the healing process. Sometimes a person needs space to deal with stress, anxiety or depression and, at other times, space to find inspiration and an alternative to feelings of melancholy. To support the healing process optimally, an assessment tool can be used to take into account salutogenic and pathogenic strategies. In addition, to ensure the satisfaction and support of different people, and to support the different phases of the healing process, the range and order of qualities (access to nature and surrounding life) is based on the challenge gradient. The challenge gradient is intended as a guide to the overall design of an enriched garden, which can help the designer to deliberately place these qualities in a way that supports the healing process.

These challenges, designed to encourage regular, spontaneous visits to nursing homes by people with Alzheimer's disease, are summed up in the following objectives of the standing invitation:

5.3. Closeness and Easy Access

The enriched garden shall be physically close to, visible and easily accessible from the spaces of the indoor environment where residents spend time. This should be the primary criteria to determine the location of the garden, particularly when considering residents with temporo-spatial disorders. It is better to choose a smaller, easily accessible parcel than a larger one that is not visible from inside and is difficult to access. This visibility of the "enriched garden" can be appreciated from the resident's bedroom window, while walking along a corridor, or from the bay windows of the living room or dining area. It also serves as a reminder of the presence of this enriched environment and supports the idea that the garden space is an integral part of the resident's living environment.

Naturally, care must be taken to ensure that the visible landscape offered by the enriched garden is aesthetically pleasing and attractive. If a resident who suffers from the heat in summer sees a garden without shade and exposed to full sun, or if he feels without being there that the garden is exposed to strong winds, or that he won't be able to find shelter there if it rains, or that he won't be able to find a place to rest, he will probably give up going there.

This garden is designed for frail people whose major fear is the risk of falling, and so this visibility from inside also addresses their fear of being isolated in the event of a problem. The fact that they can be seen and supervised from a distance by healthcare professionals is a reassuring element that helps put residents in the right mindset to visit the enriched garden on their own.

The attractiveness of the enriched garden must therefore be given particular attention by including flower beds that are visible from inside the nursing home. For this reason, it was decided that these areas should feature a rich variety of plants that changes with the seasons. It is therefore preferable to see new colors appear, with deciduous plants blooming in spring and summer, and offering colorful foliage in autumn, rather than a well-trimmed hedge of evergreens.

Similarly, different plant profiles should be formed, supported by a generous choice of ground covers, perennials, grasses and shrubs, combining a diversity of colours through foliage, flowers, bark and the presence of berries.

In order to facilitate access to the enriched garden, careful attention should be paid to all aspects of accessibility. If the garden is close and visible, it is essential to ensure easy access to it by limiting the presence of obstacles. First, we recommend that the door to the outside opens automatically and does not require an access code to be operated. If this solution is not technically possible, care should be taken to choose a door that is not too heavy to handle, and that does not close on itself too quickly. This is particularly important to make it easy for a person in a wheelchair to exit the building. As demonstrated by Cohen-Mansfield in a study assessing the limitation of access to outdoor spaces and the prevalence of disruptive behaviour disorders and depression, this door should remain unlocked if possible during the hours when residents are likely to go to the enriched garden. Among the obstacles that should be limited, it is important to remove the threshold bars under the door, as well as eliminate steps or stairs, unstable or sliding floor coverings likely to cause tripping or difficult manoeuvring, particularly for people with reduced mobility.

Designers should consider installing gates that are disguised, e.g., as part of the fence, to prevent residents with cognitive impairments from wandering outside the garden. As well as specifically designing the entrance to the garden in such a way as to reassure residents that it will be easy to reach, it is also important to signal to residents that they will have access to a pleasant space for which they will not have to make any particular arrangements., The goal is not to produce too great a contrast with the overprotected atmosphere which is generally their experience in indoor spaces.

I remember a discussion with a geriatrician, a department head in a geriatric hospital, who pointed out that caregivers generally tend to overprotect patients, especially in anticipation of a fall. She further observed that those residents going to the "enriched garden" showed themselves capable of much better balance and of stepping over small shrubs, simply because the environment had restored to them a form of confidence in their abilities and had stimulated their desire to walk there without constraints.

5.4. Attractiveness

Attractiveness is part of this notion of a permanent invitation to residents and comes in many elements that should be integrated into the design of an enriched environment. In practice, the garden space needs to integrate adapted modules which will regularly solicit the attention of the residents and make them want to visit the garden. In order to give a few examples, we cite here different types of stimulation that were implemented. They can be:

- visual: installing windmills in a mass of grasses will provide movement and contrast with the static views that the indoor environment offers. The effect of the wind on the rotation of the mills and the waving of the grass leaves create a natural dynamic that

catches the eye and produces a magical effect in the atmosphere of a garden.
- sound: installing musical instruments adapted to the external conditions gives the opportunity for residents to make music and to hear others producing melodies. On the other hand, the use of windchimes has proven to be counterproductive, because their continuous ringing as soon as there is a little wind is a source of annoyance, especially if the sound is produced in the middle of the night.
- gustatory: using edible plants - motivated quite simply by the pleasure of picking fruits from nature for yourself.

Other elements can complete this development, in particular appropriate signage to make it easy for disoriented people to find their way, and to act as a regular invitation to residents to visit the garden by reminding them of its presence and how to reach the garden. The design of this signage is very important, on the one hand because it is aimed at people potentially suffering from visual impairment (retinopathy, AMD, glaucoma), but also because this signage must not resemble too closely the style of signage commonly used in public spaces since we also wish to encourage spatial appropriation. This signage must be part of the intimate relationship that users can establish with their environment.

Many other elements could thus be set out formulating the necessary balance between freedom and security for nursing home residents. Most of our work has highlighted how necessary it is to get out of a conceptual and formatted design in order to adapt as much as possible to the capacities but also the deficiencies of vulnerable people. Finding the right balance between "the outstretched hand" to guide residents and the trap of infantilization or cliché, is a necessary exercise that will determine whether residents visit their garden regularly and appropriate it as their own space.

Many previous works have given interesting and detailed indications in this field - we will mention in particular those of Zeisel and Tyson, and Bengtsson who have developed indications relating to wayfinding for dementia and architectural adaptation for people with neurological and cognitive disorders. Other publications present lists of good ideas for the arrangement of space but which are unfortunately also overbearing in terms of social constructs and cultural heritage. We will thus cite the regular temptation to install water features and fountains based on ideas that we have about the effect of the sound of running water to help anxious people feel serene and peaceful. This is undoubtedly true, but in practice the running water, especially in summer, will be a continuous temptation for confused residents to come and quench their thirst, which imposes the difficult task on the nursing home management of guaranteeing that this water is always drinkable. Moreover, we must consider the effect that the sound of water may produce on people suffering from incontinence.

The objective of this work is not to become a guide for the construction of an enriched garden, but above all to make visible the complete paradigm shift that this approach requires. Creating an enriched garden involves developing the environment and designing it from a human-centred perspective, whereas landscape designers have been trained and work essentially to develop the environment based on its climatic, spatial, agronomic, and geographical characteristics, and then inserting ideas, representations and symbols intended to sensitise and move visitors.

The framework used in the design of enriched gardens is only part of an intermediate and experimental phase of transposing the concept of an enriched environment to humans and then undertaking its extension to all their living spaces in order to establish a salutogenic vision while, of course, also respecting the environment and biodiversity.

Such a logic only makes sense if it can be validated scientifically by implementing robust study protocols. We may also explore what the layout of the interior space will be, as well as that of more open spaces such as a village square, a town centre or the headquarters of a company. Such spaces will then be frequented by individuals with very different health profiles. This chapter gives an overview of this deployment of the enriched environment in our places of life based on the experiences accumulated by our research work.

6. The Enrichment of the Enriched Garden

The principle of enriching garden spaces was inspired by research on the enriched environment. It has been adapted to take into account the specificities of life in nursing homes and Alzheimer's disease.

We grounded this design work in a constructivist approach, and it was an important part of the development of the enriched gardens. Following the pragmatic thought expressed by Lapoujade (169), *"Trust does not consist in carrying out an action whose success is assured, but in attempting an action whose outcome is uncertain."* Lechopier [170] reformulates it this way: *"We must remain attentive to the unexpected, to what remains in motion: thought is a distributed practice, not the contemplation by a scientist of eternal truths."* It is in this spirit that each of the enrichment modules was subjected to an evaluation as part of a pilot phase for which accessibility, appropriation and intuitive interaction with the resident were evaluated. Depending on the results of this evaluation, we subjected the modules to a series of complementary cycles of optimization and adjustments.

About fifty different enrichment modules have thus been designed and adapted according to the therapeutic objectives envisaged for an enriched garden project. Following the assessment of the main health issues that have been identified among the nursing home residents, a combination of these modules makes it possible to give an enriched garden priority for one or more of the following targets:

- Behavioural problems
- Functional autonomy
- Cognitive disorders: temporal-spatial orientation, procedural memory, circadian rhythm, executive functions, praxis
- Prevention of falls: walking, balance
- Motor skills and fine motor skills
- Social connections
- Mood disorders: depression, self-esteem

6.1. Serenity Space

The serenity space is formed by a line of wooden poles and architectural plants. It is open on a double layer translucide screen forming continuous wave movements.

It creates a soothing envelope which is both open and closed. Sitting on a bench in this space is intended to soothe behavioural disorders (Photography 1).

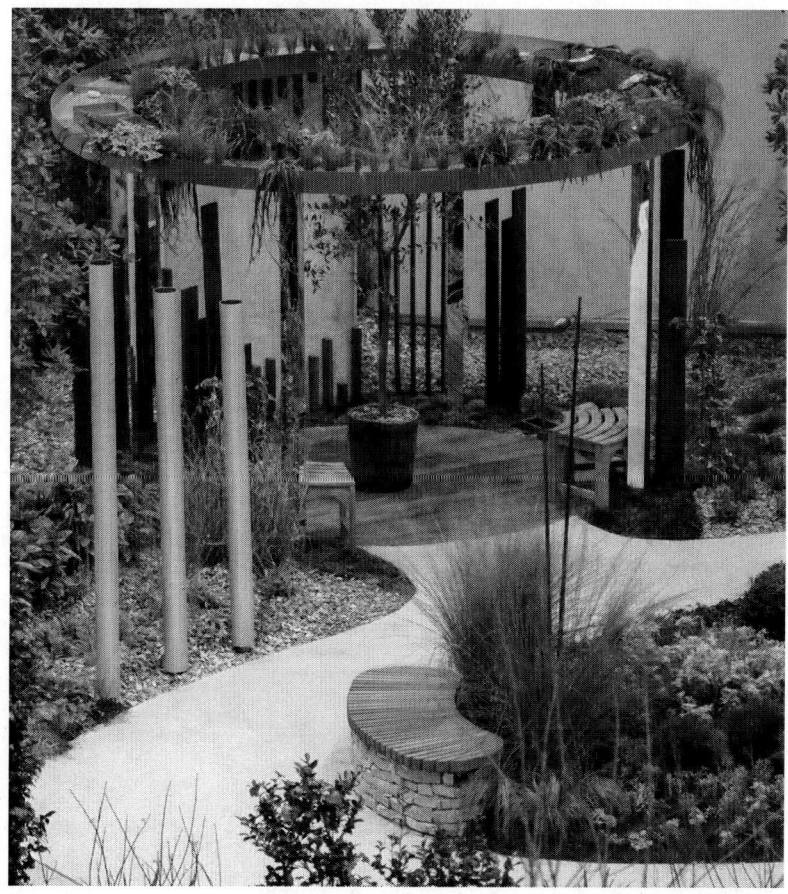

Photograph 1. Serenity space at a Landscaping exhibition in Lyon (France) 2017.

6.2. Garden Easel

This is an outdoor easel intended to receive painting expressions. Leave the trace of a gesture, and express an emotion with a brush stroke. These paint lines wash away with rain (or a sponge) and create an emotional and cognitive connection with the landscape. Residents can paint with a brush or with their fingers.

The presence of the easel in the garden is part of the residents' journey from being from spectators to being actors in their environment. Painting on the easel can be a spontaneous action when visiting the garden or can be part of a workshop activity (Photography 2).

The gesture of the brush dipped in one of the pots of colour will leave an imprint on the landscape. There is no issue of success or failure in the practice of this brush stroke. This transition to a proactive relationship in the garden underlined by the imprint on the canvas stimulates emotional perception and encourages voluntary praxis.

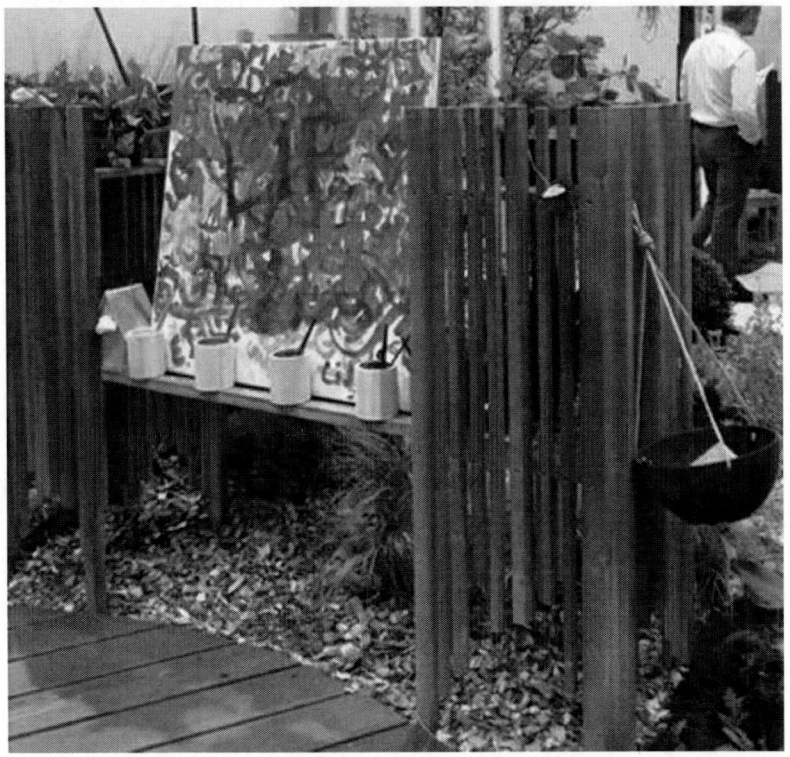

Photograph 2. Garden easel at a Landscaping exhibition in Lyon (France) 2017.

6.3. Sensory Stimulation Amplification Pyramid

This module is designed in a pyramidal structure producing an ordered association of sensory stimulations. It offers a range of materials, colors, smells, sounds and amplified tastes to stimulate the senses. The resident can interact with a cascade of plants whose sensation to the touch gradually evolves from the roughest to the silkiest (Photography 3). Likewise, for tastes, the plants present a variety ranging from sweet to acidic, the smells range from the most to the least fragrant, and visually, the carpet of plants progresses from dark to lighter colors. The layout of the activity area is defined structurally by the materials used (wood, stone…), with the colors and the aromas and an association of the senses on several levels, and with exploratory sensory games.

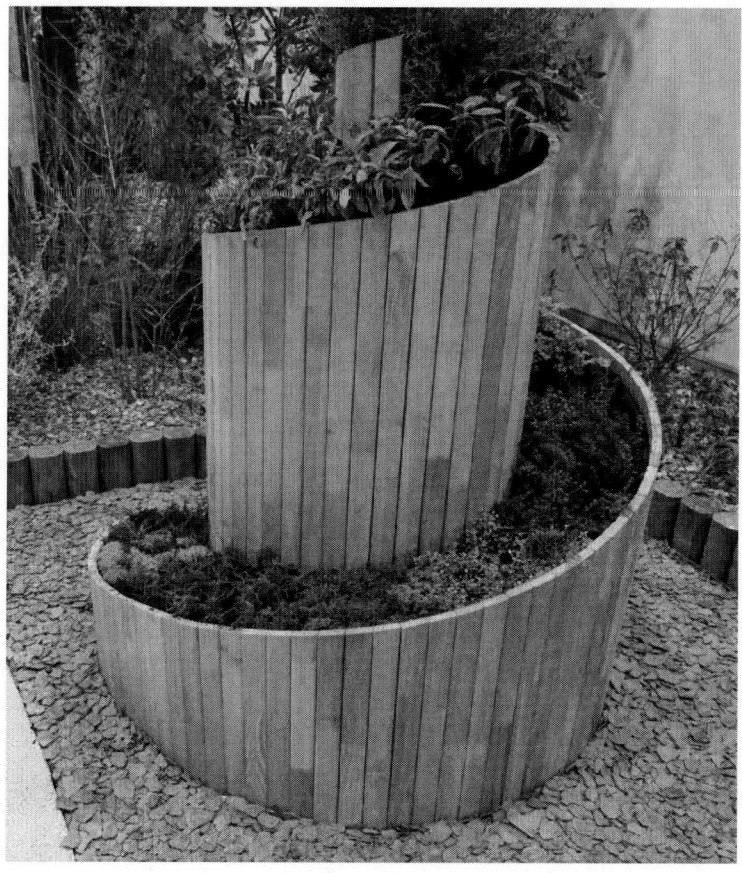

Photograph 3. Sensory pyramid at a Landscaping exhibition in Lyon (France) 2017.

6.4. Garden Sundial

This module is formed by a sundial which shows the resident's shadow projected onto a circle or plants arranged in sections matching the colors of the rainbow. As the resident views her shadow projected from the base of the sundial she is given an indication of temporality – represented by a symbol recalling the main activities of the day (Photography 4).

This notion of temporality fixed by the colors of the rainbow is taken up in a spatial dimension by stepping stones in the same colors making a path across the enriched garden. We saw that when we moved the stepping stones to form a different path, the majority of residents with major neurocognitive disorders followed the new path spontaneously without however having received any verbal instructions.

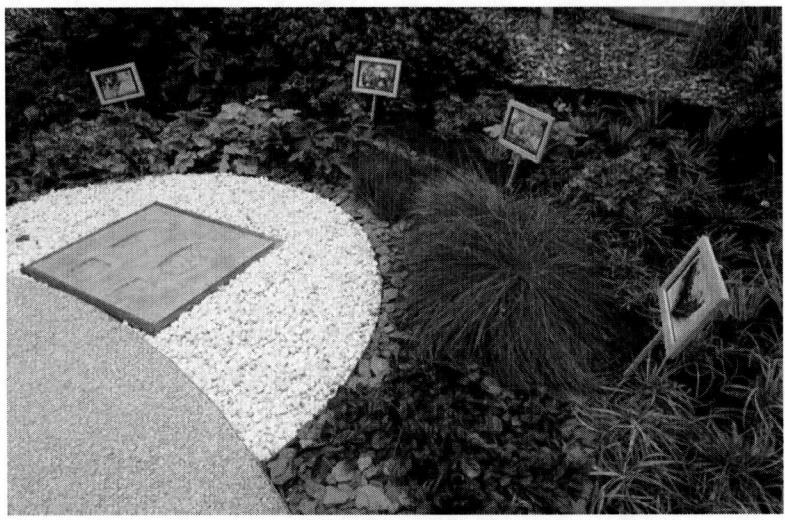

Photograph 4. Garden sundial at a Landscaping exhibition in Lyon (France) 2017.

6.5. Floor Painting

This module is intended to produce traces of paint on the ground from a large, movable brush hanging from a cable that is stretched over a length of 3 meters. The resident moves the brush over a surface designed to receive the paint, which flows onto it by gravity. The resident holds on to the brush using two "bicycle handlebar grip"-type handles. The fresh paint comes from a bucket of paint in which the resident has previously dipped the brush. Inherited from calligraphy, the practice of painting by gravity (vertical flow) is a vector for the expression and translation of the painter's emotions that are made visible by the line of the paint on the floor surface. This paint disappears with the rain or can be wiped away with squeegee.

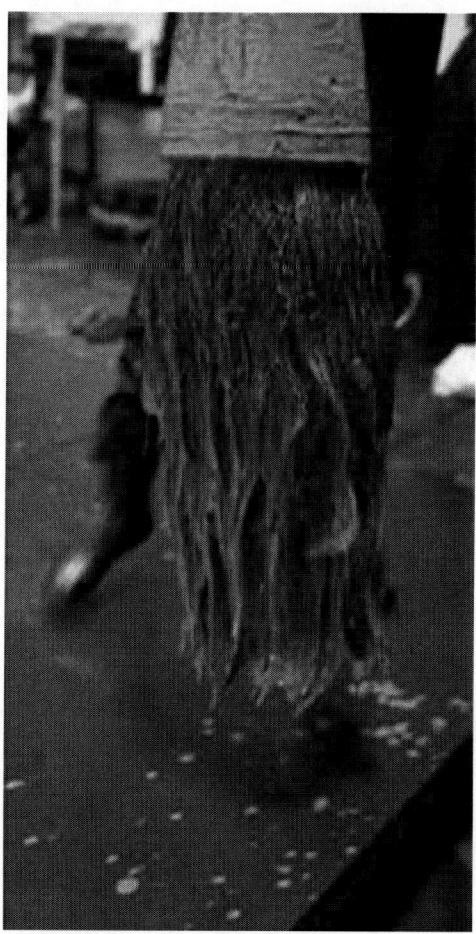

Photograph 5. Floor painting.

Inspired by the visionary artist Fabienne Verdier, this module came into being after we made adaptations for the specific ergonomic and functional needs of the older adults. It serves as a real tool for liberation and spatial appropriation while promoting the emotional expression of anxiety disorders (Photography 5).

6.6. Gardening Corner

Integrating gardening activity into an enriched garden was originally a necessity as it seemed to flow naturally.

We made a crucial choice to avoid the use of raised beds which are generally unattractive and above all reinforce the artificiality of the garden space, instead of offering visitors a more intimate relationship with nature.

In our space, gardening activity is suggested and facilitated but it is certainly not obligatory. The working group underlined how little time nursing home's residents spend gardening. It was a question of reinventing "gardening" by giving it a playful form and by freeing itself from the temporality which presents too great a constraint. This is especially true for people suffering from dementia and who find it difficult to get involved in the time between planting, the emergence of young shoots and the production of flowers or fruits. The ergonomic gardening corner is intended to accompany the relief, profile and shapes of the garden.

Furthermore, it has been observed that residents from a rural background do not always enjoy gardening, which they associate with doing chores; while for others from an urban environment, the aspiration to garden proved to be far removed from their preoccupation. This activity area weaves a physical link with nature and the plant - but it reverses the traditional image of the garden perceived as a "workplace" by retaining only the playful and artistic dimension. We identified these key criteria:

- Adapt the ergonomics of the garden.
- Integrate workstations with accessibility for people with reduced mobility into the ergonomic embankment.
- Adapt the dimensions of the embankment (height, depth), the materials used according to the soil, the vegetation according to the proposed activities.

Sculpture and plant weaving:

People can form braids and shapes with long grasses using their hands.. This activity is both creative and/or uses procedural memory.

- Amplify sensory stimulation on the talus.

6.7. Musical Instruments

We worked with a British instrumentalist who specialises in the design of music tools that are suitable for outdoor use to create a set of musical instruments, including the Rainbow Xylophone, that can be set up in an enriched garden (Photography 6). The Rainbow Xylophone allows the player to express themselves spontaneously through a set of hammers attached to the instrument. They can also play a melody figured on a score represented by colored notes or by copying a rhythm supported by another instrument, a song or a soundtrack. The design of this instrument invites varied fine motor work depending on the horizontal or vertical layout of the xylophone.

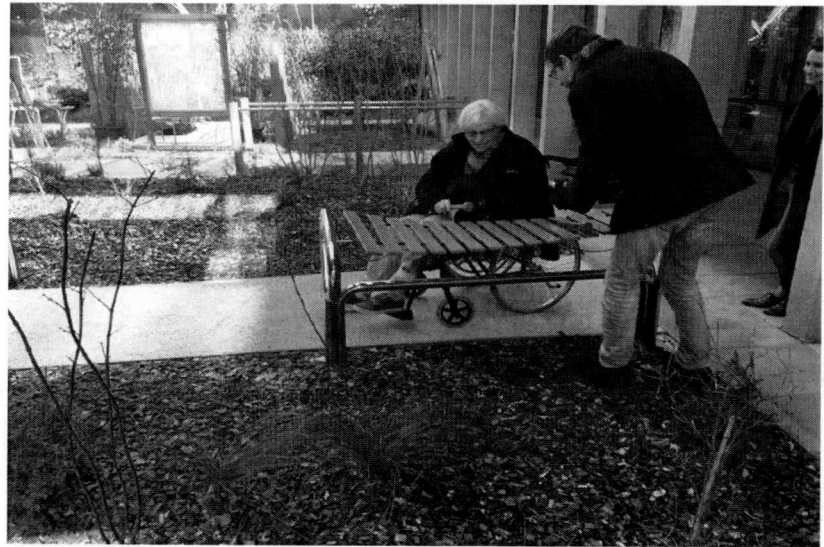

Photograph 6. Outdoor musical instruments in nursing homes.

Chapter 6

Philosophical Background and Currents of Thought

1. Major Philosophical Theories Supporting the Enriched Environment

Two philosophical currents offer competing responses. Weber [171] and Boudon [172], taking a methodological individualist approach, propose a response that considers "*the isolated individual and his activity, and not the group, as the basic unit of comprehensive sociology, I would say its atom.*"

By analyzing human behaviour, Boudon [173] defends the autonomy of the individual in his or her choices and beliefs. At the other end of the spectrum is Bourdieu's vision [174], which he summarised in his latest book, "*Les Méditations pascaliennes.*" Bourdieu's structuralist approach considers that the individual is the product of social constructs, from which he or she cannot escape. Through their habitus - the rules they have assimilated - people make their choices and take their actions through the intermediary of the collective structures with which they are imbued. For Bourdieu, the individual cannot be separated from society. In the context of our research, these two visions offer a very different analysis of the relationship that an nursing home resident will establish with a garden. Bourdieu's approach is that there is no standard garden, no standard physical environment, and that the design of the garden must take account of each person's habitus - i.e., their background (socio-professional, rural or urban) and their level of education. Boudon takes into account the consciousness of the individual.

Boudon believes that, rather than Bourdieu's social determinism, each person has the ability to make choices based on his or her background. In this case, when it comes to appreciating a garden or the physical environment of a nursing home, the resident is not necessarily going to look for what best reflects the social constructs of the environment from which he or she comes. For Boudon, it is not a question of offering a resident from a well-off, highly educated background a garden that corresponds to the stereotype of his or her class. We usually assume that a nursing home resident from a rural background will feel much more at home in a garden than a city dweller. Conversely, we often see people from large urban centres actively seeking proximity to nature, explaining that they have been deprived of it. Do we need to look to the past for the reasons why each individual visits a garden, as Weber and Boudon advocate, or is there a social determinism that motivates their practice, as Bourdieu proposes? The way to reconcile these two currents is to consider a conception of the physical environment based on habitus, and then to draw on detailed survey work derived from Dewey's social constructivism [175], to identify the residents' expectations more precisely.

The environment, when it refers to nature through the garden, is framed by numerous conceptual frameworks. Bergson's creative evolution [176] invites us to approach nature as an explanation and support for the élan vital (his terminology). Latour's approach [177] to the sociology of science offers a vision of nature built on a distinction between human and non-human. Latour describes it as an ontology with variable geometry, depending on whether we consider nature to be a human construct responding to societal expectations or a rule of nature. Following this, Descola [178] rejects the idea that "there is a single nature and plural cultures, which would be guilty of ethnocentrism, given that the nature supposedly standing behind all cultures is none other than that defined by our science, i.e., a product of our culture." In his work, Descola has endeavoured to "*demonstrate the prevalence of a naturalist ontology, specific to Western societies, which presents a worldview opposing the concepts of nature and culture in the constitution of science.*" This duality explains and justifies the duality between social anthropology and physical anthropology.

Descola [179] adds in his plea: "It's time to answer a possible question. Where do you fit into the great debate between universalism and relativism? How can you at once challenge the generality of the distinction between nature and culture and claim to uncover invariants in the ways in which humans relate to non-humans?" Our enriched garden, in this respect, lies on the fragile fringe between non-human nature and human constructs. Some see it as a representation of nature, while others recognise it as a representation of the human ideal. In his concept of the ecumene, Berque [180] developed that "man cannot live without a place, without a qualification of space," and that this milieu - the ecumene - is formed by the relationship that the individual establishes with space and nature. According to Berque, this relationship exists on multiple levels. It is ecological, symbolic and technological - this triptych constituting the anthropisation of the Earth. Berque [181] emphasises the extent to which this relationship is born of experience. An individual's understanding of his or her environment is based on the actions and gestures that, in a given space and culture, shape this experience.

These interactions between nature and mankind raise questions about their direct or indirect effects on human health. Does the beneficial effect of the environment on health resonate with the place and order reserved for it by man? To explain this, should we, as Latour [182] suggests, descend into the earth's "burning pits" to study "*the fires that animate it*" and analyse the origin of the effects it can produce on humans?

Does the assertion that nature and gardens are the ideal environment for restoring health and well-being, as made in the Barnes, Cooper Marcus and Hartig studies [182, 183, 184], apply to all humans who frequent nature and gardens? Do we see differences in effects and efficiency on different people, and if so, on what basis are these differences in interaction with the environment established? Returning to gardens and nature, the Boudonian approach suggests that there is an explanation for each individual's attraction or reluctance to frequent them, and that the relationship that a person establishes with his environment should be read in the light of his own consciousness and past experiences. How can we apply a collective vision of the action of the environment, when each individual develops his or her own experience of it? Our analysis leads to a more complex understanding, combining each individual's choice based on his or her own experience and social constructs, with the influence of the environment in which these people live. The design, general architecture and accessibility of enriched gardens all contribute to how well they are used. Exposure to an enriched garden compensates for the "impoverished" environment of some nursing homes.

This questioning resonates with the "oxygen bubble" that a garden represents in relation to the physical environment of a nursing home. This understanding of the role of enriched gardens also requires us to take into account the health of residents, their frailties, their disorders and chronic pathologies. The associated question is to assess the influence of their general condition on their ability to visit and participate in the life of the enriched garden. This ability to visit a garden results from the interaction between the resident's self-perception and how attractive they find the garden. This dimension of interest is described by the concept of appropriation of space by the user.

2. Scientific Relativism

Should the health effects of a garden be assessed in response to the social construct of the garden, or within the framework of a scientific approach? This question calls into question the choice of scientific methodology. Popper's critical rationalism [185] defines the need for a scientific approach whose results are validated by the exercise of refutation. As Popper writes: "does science place itself in the expectation of knowledge that is a little truer, more universal and more complete, or is it ready for a refutation of existing knowledge by an experiment that would dethrone it?" Popper's reflections led him to question the validity of an inductive approach in scientific research, so much so that he proposed as a criterion of a theory's scientificity "the possibility of invalidating, refuting or testing it." In this respect, theories based on one-off experiments, such as Ulrich's hospital windows opening onto trees, should be compared with the "universal" theory that nature heals and potentially cures.

Wittgenstein's scientific relativism suggests that the conclusions of scientific work cannot rationally be extended to all situations that come close to them - thus criticizing a mythology of the rule.

Alternatively, Latour proposes a pragmatic constructivism, drawing jointly on scientific methodology and the human sciences. For Latour, there is no such thing as a single scientific method, since hypotheses and their interpretation are the result of social construction. Where there is a single criterion of rationality for Popper, there are multiple criteria of rationality for Latour. Latour's approach to this research suggests combining a rigorous methodology for assessing the effectiveness of the enriched garden on nursing home residents, with a survey strategy that gathers the behaviours and perceptions of the garden's stakeholders - caregivers, residents, carers - in order to measure the potential controversies that exist around the assessment criteria in what Latour calls "the court of reason."

This ontological picture is shaped by conflicts and contradictions between currents. It serves to keep a critical eye on the choices and analyses made by practitioners. This is true of Bourdieu's approach, which is opposed to Boudon's, and also of Latour's vision of nature between the human and the non-human. In the relationship that the older adults establish with their environment, it is important to assess which part of social determinism or individualism predominates.

This vision of centring the environment in order to satisfy human health reinforces an anthropomorphic conception of nature, which is certainly the opposite of Descola's approach which encourages breaking with this constant distinction between human and non-human.

The salutogenic vision promoted by the enriched environment is consequently at a crossroads - inviting us to question the anthropomorphic reading of the world, as suggested by many ethnologists and anthropologists, and finally, as Descola sums up: *"What is being questioned is not the form of the dualistic opposition, but the universality of the content that has been attributed to some of them, such as the opposition between nature and culture."*

In terms of therapeutic practices, public health policies have been based on rational processes likely to produce reliable and repeatable scientific results. The fact that enriched environments have been studied mainly in the context of basic research by neurobiologists, rather than clinicians, may partly explain the absence of solid experience in transposing these principles to humans. Nevertheless, the richness of the environment is relative by virtue of the different social environments in which humans exist, and the many uncontrollable variables in the environment. Moreover, stimulating EE patterns are not always easy to control. In addition, stimulating EE patterns are codetermined by the patient's choice, according to his or her interests and the specific environment of a medical-social establishment, whether a geriatric hospital or a nursing home. This understanding of the interaction between an individual and his or her environment according to his or her own social constructs is therefore a decisive element in advancing the use and democratization of enriched environments as a health practice for humans.

3. Impoverished Environments

Contrary to enriched environments, Donald Hebb also described the concept of impoverished environments. Without mentioning the controversy over Hebb's work with the CIA and torture [186], it is essential to understand the different gradients of environmental enrichment and how these are reflected in the reality of our living environments.

We are regularly tempted to think that the hospital environment or that of nursing homes is similar to a form of impoverished environment. What about the living environment of the inhabitants of megacities such as London, Paris, New York, Tokyo or Shanghai?

A Canadian journalist, R Louv, recently took up the question by describing nature deficit syndrome [187].

The causes of this syndrome are multiple but are essentially linked to the way of life that has developed over the last decades. Louv sums up this evolution with the following sentence "the parents had grown up in nature, while their children grew up in the house."

Among the first predictors of nature deficit syndrome is the development of a sedentary lifestyle. Over the past 30 years, the amount of territory on which children can move and play without the direct supervision of their parents has decreased by 90%. This is associated with the explosion in the use of new technologies, which are an additional enticement for children (and adults) not to leave their homes.

Another element concerns the development of the territories (of which green spaces and sustainable architecture are major issues) and the opportunities for immersion.

Nature deficit syndrome is a particularly significant syndrome for young people with multiple disabilities who, in the course of their lives and their learning, have regularly been deprived of contact with nature because of their disability. Moving around in a shell chair, a child with motor challenges may have even less experience with nature than city children, who have had very little opportunity or even no opportunity at all to have leaves, earth, moss or pine cones in their hands. According to Dr. Melissa Lem, family physician, faculty member in the Department of Family and Community Medicine at the University of Toronto and member of the Canadian Association of Physicians for the Environment: *"Spending time in nature is essential for the proper development of a child, psychologically as well as physically. Some researchers even claim that a daily dose of nature can prevent and treat many medical conditions."*

She cites studies on, for example:

- Attention deficit hyperactivity disorder (ADHD): 5 to 10% of children in Canada
- Weight gain and obesity: one in four Canadian children
- High blood pressure, diabetes and cholesterol-related problems on the rise among young Canadians
- Myopia, asthma, depression
- Delays in the development of motor skills and social skills

This reading of the nature deficit syndrome would lead us to understand what for each is an acceptable definition of nature. I have had the opportunity to hear two very different perceptions of a traditional Auvergne landscape in central France, where Charolais cattle were peacefully grazing - some exclaiming enthusiastically: "It's nice to be able to get back in touch with nature!" and the others facing the same landscape saying despairingly: "It's sad to see all these meat factories!"

Will an enriched environment for some people be considered a normal environment for others? This is what we have tried to assess in the studies that we present to you in the following chapters. We include a quantitative study on the effects of an enriched environment on a population of people with advanced Alzheimer's disease and living in nursing homes, and a qualitative study on spatial appropriation by residents also living with Alzheimer's disease in nursing homes.

Chapter 7

Enriched Environments: Potential Benefits for Human Health

1. The First Transposition Study of Enriched Environment in Geriatric Institution

The effects of enriched environments have been studied in several animal studies, but very few models have been transposed to humans according to the principles of translational research.

However, it is not known whether an enriched environment would have a positive effect on people with dementia. The design and implementation of enriched gardens within nursing homes was designed to be a candidate for translational research on enriched environments and the evaluation of the benefits of an enriched environment on residents with Alzheimer's disease. To address this question, we designed a cluster pilot trial to determine whether environmental enrichment applied to nursing home gardens could have beneficial effects on clinical markers of functioning in residents with dementia.

1.1. Settings

This multicentre, cluster-controlled pilot trial was carried out in four French nursing homes that had both a conventional sensory garden and an enriched garden designed by a specialised landscape architect [92]. These four nursing homes were selected to take part in the study because they all had both an enriched garden and a conventional sensory garden, which is not a common situation. We obtained a list of nursing homes where enriched gardens had been installed in recent years by asking garden design companies. We contacted the nursing homes to find out whether they also had a conventional sensory garden and whether access was separate from their enriched garden. Finally, we asked the directors of these establishments if they would be interested in taking part in the study. The outdoor gardens were separate and had specific access points, with no possibility of moving directly from one garden to the other. The gardens were open to residents during the day and closed at night.

Garden enrichment is the result of specific research and design ideas to create facilities adapted to the implementation of therapeutic objectives. Each enriched garden module was the result of a collaborative design process with several staff members and teams of architects. Table 1 shows the types of activities or environments implemented in the enriched gardens and the designers' objectives. The enriched garden's activity areas and special environments were designed for intuitive use, without special written or oral instructions or human facilitation. Enriched garden areas ranged from 300 to 600 square meters.

We present tables below highlighting the distribution of the different gardens within the nursing homes.

In each nursing home, we defined three sectors corresponding to care units. Depending on the location and proximity of the gardens, one sector was considered to be close to the enriched garden, another close to the sensory garden, and the last unit was not close to any garden. Participants were assigned to one of the three groups according to the location of their rooms in these sectors.

Residents in these areas were eligible for the study if they had Alzheimer's disease or another type of dementia and were able to walk independently without human assistance. The diagnosis of Alzheimer's disease or another type of dementia was made by the facility's general practitioner and/or medical coordinator and was specifically mentioned in the resident's medical record. Patients with severe cognitive impairment, defined as MMSE<10 (Mini Mental Status Examination), and patients with severe behavioural disorders were excluded. All eligible residents were invited to take part in the study and were assigned to one of three groups according to the location of their room in the units: Conventional Garden Group, Enriched Garden Group or Control Group.

1.2. Intervention

The interventions took place over six months, in spring and summer. For participants in the "conventional sensory garden" and "enriched garden" groups, the intervention aimed to encourage them to visit their assigned garden frequently. For participants in the control group, usual care was applied and no specific intervention was carried out to encourage them to visit the gardens.

For the conventional sensory garden group, we asked staff members in their unit to remind and invite participants to visit the conventional sensory garden. We asked them to do this several times a day, so as to achieve four visits per week per participant. We also asked staff members to accompany residents to the entrance of the garden and encourage them to walk around. Residents would usually stroll through the garden on their own or with other residents for 10 to 20 minutes, and we did not ask staff to accompany them when they visited the garden. Staff members were also asked to invite families to use the corresponding garden with their family member.

For the enriched garden group, we asked staff members in their unit to remind and invite participants to visit the enriched garden, with the same recommendations regarding the frequency of visits.

In addition, shortly after recruiting the participants, the healthcare professionals were given the task of introducing the "enriched garden" enrichment modules to each resident in this group, during a short individual visit lasting around 15 minutes. Then, over the following months, each resident had his or her own interaction experience with the modules, being free to develop interactions according to his or her own intuition. The route through the garden from one visit to the next could be different, with the resident not necessarily stopping at the same stations each time.

For the control group, we didn't give staff members any instructions about visiting the gardens, and they in turn did not give these residents any specific requests to visit the gardens. It was observed that without these regular invitations from the caregivers, participants in the control group made very few, if any, visits to the gardens.

During the study, free access to the gardens was provided by doors that opened and unlocked automatically from 8 a.m. to 8 p.m., and access to the gardens was not restricted to anyone in the facility. This meant that all residents could visit any garden, whether or not they were participating in the study, and whatever group they were assigned to.

Of course, visitors and residents' families were welcome to accompany residents in the gardens.

1.3. Training the Health Professionals

Before starting the study and implementing the interventions, we organised two two-hour meetings for all staff members, regardless of the units in which they worked. In each of the four nursing homes, 10 to 12 staff members attended one of these meetings. At these meetings, one of us presented the aim of the study and the role of staff members in implementing the interventions, namely to encourage participants assigned to either the conventional sensory garden or the enriched garden to visit their respective gardens (conventional sensory garden and enriched garden) at least four times a week, and also to ensure that residents visited their gardens regularly. We did not instruct staff members to accompany residents to the garden and spend time with them. With the exception of a few specific activities, most resident visits took place without professional assistance.

1.4. Measures

For participating residents at each facility, two observers (a psychologist and an occupational therapist), independent of the research team, performed the following assessments at baseline and after six months:

- Global cognitive function using the Mini Mental Status Examination (MMSE). The MMSE is an evaluation scale regularly used in geriatrics intended to evaluate the evolution of a patient's cognitive abilities from an "initial cognitive capital" that each person has since birth. In the case of people with major neurocognitive disorders (e.g., Alzheimer's disease, dementia with Lewy bodies) a loss of 1 to 2 MMSE points per year is observed depending on the progression of the disease.
- Level of independence using activities of daily living (ADL). This evaluation scale is a relevant indicator of the evolution of the independence of people and in particular of the older adults. The loss of autonomy is a significant marker of a person's ability to carry out the actions of daily life on their own. The inability to accomplish essential activities of daily living may lead to unsafe conditions and poor quality of life. Measuring an individual's ADLs is important because they are predictors of admission to nursing homes, need for alternative living arrangements, hospitalisation, use of paid home

care, and level necessary care of the resident by the institution. Major neurocognitive disorders, including Alzheimer's disease, cause continuous and generally irreversible damage to functional independence.
- Risk of falls were measured with gait and balance tests using the Timed Up and Go test (TUG) and Unipodal stance tests respectively.
- The TUG test measures a time value in seconds, quantifying the time necessary for the participant to perform the test. This goes as follows (the higher the value, the higher the risk of falling):
  - Patients wear their usual shoes and can use a walking aid if needed.
  - The patient starts in a sitting position
  - The patient gets up at the command of the therapist, walks 5 metres, turns around, returns to the chair and sits down.
  - Time stops when the patient is seated.
- The Unipodal Stance test or Single Leg Stance (SLS) is used to assess static postural and balance control. Combined with the TUG test, these tests are significant predictors of the risk of falling and can help to monitor neurological and psychomotricity conditions. This test measures a value in seconds and is performed as follows: (The lower the value, the higher the risk of falling).
  - Performed with eyes open and hands on the hips.
  - Patient stands on one leg unassisted; time begins when the opposite foot leaves the ground; time stops immediately when the opposite foot touches the ground and/or when hands leave the hips.

The evaluators did not receive a description of the protocol. They therefore assessed each participant without knowing the purpose of the study and the participant's allocated group, in accordance with the blinded assessment process.

We did not measure the time spent by residents in the gardens. Also, we are unable to accurately describe the percentage of time when residents used the gardens independently. On average, each nursing home had staff-led activities in the gardens (approximately 45 min) twice a month mostly between May and early September. Thus, most of the time spent by residents in the gardens was done without the presence of staff members.

1.5. Participants

Of the 368 residents at the four facilities, 220 (60%) had been diagnosed with Alzheimer's disease or another type of dementia, and 266 (72%) were able to walk on their own. A total of 140 residents were included in the study after selecting eligible participants from the four nursing homes. Seventeen dropouts occurred during the 6 months of follow-up, including 6 in the control group, 5 in the conventional sensory garden group and 6 in the enriched garden group. These dropouts were the result of events that occurred during the trial, such as hospitalisation and loss of independent walking. Data was missing for 3 residents and these data were not included in the final results. Thus, the data of 120 residents were analysed, including 39 residents of the control group, 41 residents of the conventional sensory garden group and 40 residents of the enriched garden group (Figure 13).

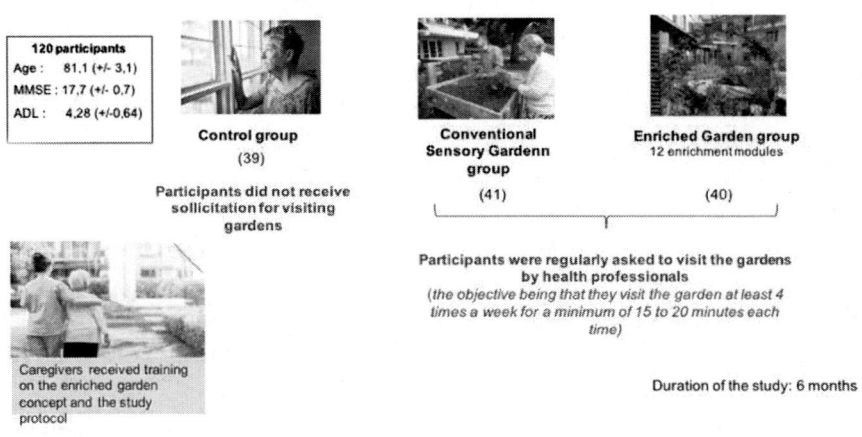

Figure 13. Quantitative longitudinal interventional study summary protocol.

The residents' characteristics in each group are shown in the table below. No significant differences were observed between the three groups in age, gender, baseline MMSE, ADL, TUG or unipodal stance values. The setting characteristics reflect the distribution of participants among the four nursing homes participating in this study (Table 3).

Table 3. Participants characteristics

	Control group (n=39)	Conventional sensory gardens group (n=41)	Enriched garden group (n=40)	P value
Age (years)	81·1 +/- 3·5	80·5 +/- 3·6	80·9 +/- 3·5	0·70
Sex				
% of women	26 (67%)	28 (68%)	29 (72%)	0·81
Multicentric setting Nursing home distribution				
1	12 (31%)	10 (24%)	7 (18%)	0·93
2	8 (21%)	10 (24%)	9 (23%)	
3	13 (33%)	16 (39%)	17 (43%)	
4	6 (15%)	5 (12%)	7 (18%)	
MMSE score (0-30)	17·3 +/- 3·3	17·8 +/- 2·9	18·0 +/- 2·7	0·57
ADL (0-6)	4·28 +/- 0·69	4·29 +/- 0·66	4·27 +/- 0·54	0·98
3 ADLs	10 (25%)	8 (19%)	6 (15%)	0·37
4 ADLs	17 (44%)	20 (49%)	26 (65%)	
5 ADLs	12 (31%)	13 (32%)	8 (20%)	
Unipodal stance (sec)	8·03 +/- 4·23	8·85 +/- 4·67	8·65 +/- 4·60	0·70
< 5 sec.	10 (26%)	10 (24%)	10 (25%)	0·91
5 to 10 sec.	17 (43%)	15 (37%)	14 (35%)	
>10 sec.	12 (31%)	16 (39%)	16 (40%)	
Time up and go (sec)	15·69 +/- 4·54	14·54 +/- 3·81	15·53 +/- 5·24	0·47
< 15 sec.	14 (36%)	22 (54%)	20 (50%)	0·11
15 to 20 sec.	15 (38%)	16 (39%)	10 (25%)	
>20 sec.	10 (26%)	3 (7%)	10 (25%)	

During the 6-month follow-up, we observed a functional decline in the conventional sensory garden and control groups in MMSE, ADL, TUG and unipodal stance values. However, significant and positive effects on MMSE, ADL, TUG and unipodal stance values were observed in the enriched garden participants (see table above: Participants characteristics). The percentages of residents with improvements in independence, TUG and unipodal stance values were significantly greater in the enriched garden group compared to the two other groups (see table above: Participants characteristics). We did not record any adverse events related to garden use.

1.6. Results

This pilot study showed that incentives for nursing home residents with dementia to attend an enriched garden contributed to better functioning compared to residents who were invited to visit a conventional sensory garden or who did not visit any garden. The concept of enriched environments placed in gardens for Alzheimer's disease patients is a new approach to improve the functioning of patients with dementia.

The results of this clinical study are very promising. It showed the significant effect of enriched environment overall health indicators with an improvement of health functions as regards to cognition, risk of falls, functional independence. These simultaneous improvements of this range in geriatric clinical trials, and a fortiori in patients with advanced Alzheimer's disease, are sufficiently rare for us not to refrain from highlighting them as genuine advances in the management of dementia (Figure 14 and Table 4).

Table 4. Results of a 6 months exposure to enriched environment for nursing home residents with Alzheimer's disease (advanced stage), compared to normal environment and control group

	Control group (n=39)	Conventional sensory garden group (n=41)	Enriched garden group (n=40)	P value
Evolution of cognition measured with: MMSE Score	-0.25 +/- 0.71	-0.24 +/- 0.73	+0.93 +/- 0.65	0.0001
Evolution of Independence measured with ADL	-0.05 +/- 0.32	-0.12 +/- 0.24	0.30 +/- 0.35	0.0001
Worsen (-1)	5 (13%)	9 (22%)	1 (2%)	<0.0001
No change	30 (77%)	32 (78%)	18 (45%)	
Improved (+1)	4 (10%)	0	21 (53%)	
Evolution of risk of falls measured with:				
Unipodal stance (sec)	-1.10 +/- 2.09	-0.46 +/- 3.49	+1.78 +/- 3.84	0.0007
Worsen	39 (100%)	15 (37%)	0	<0.0001
No change	0	16 (39%)	0	
Improved	0	10 (24%)	40 (100%)	
Timed Up and Go (sec)	+0.77 +/- 2.71	+0.51 +/- 3.17	-1.95 +/- 2.98	0.0001
Worsen	15 (38%)	18 (44%)	5 (12%)	<0.0001
No change	17 (44%)	15 (37%)	14 (35%)	
Improved	7 (18%)	8 (19%)	21 (53%)	

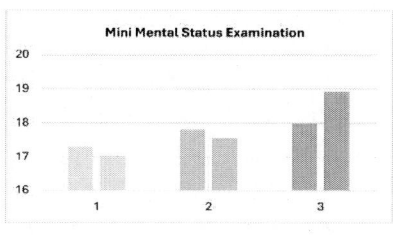
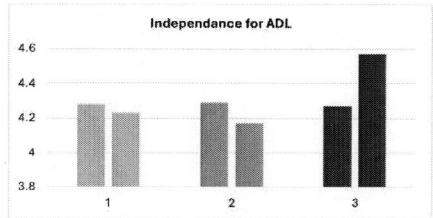
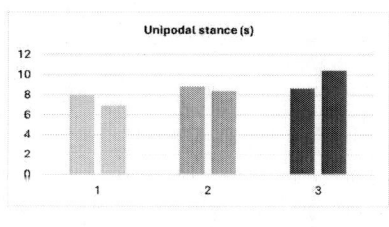
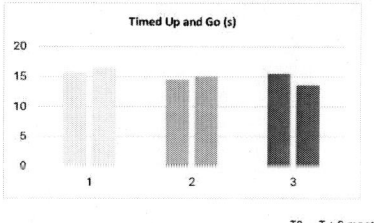

1 = Control group   2 = Visiting Conventional Sensory Garden   3 = Visiting Enriched Garden

Figure 14. Results of a longitudinal controlled multicentric study on the effects of Enriched gardens on nursing homes residents with Alzheimer's disease.

1.7. Discussion

Although previous studies highlighted the beneficial contribution of gardens to patients with Alzheimer's disease, none used a robust study protocol. This led Whear [188], who published a systematic review in 2014 to assess the effects of gardens on the health of nursing home residents with dementia, to conclude that weak study protocols made it impossible to draw clear conclusions about the benefits of gardens. None of these studies included the notion of an enriched garden. They identified ten quantitative studies, all with methodological limitations and a high risk of bias. The gardens in these studies were not specially designed for nursing home residents with dementia. Further in their scoping review, Howarth [158] identified 14 studies evaluating the effects of gardens on patients with dementia and concluded that they contributed to positive effects on disruptive behaviours and improved quality of life, but also noted that the protocols of these studies were not strong enough to present evidence.

These conclusions converge with the previous observations that we have summarised in relation to studies on the environment and health.

Our study on the effects of enriched gardens on nursing home residents with Alzheimer's disease is original and innovative in several aspects. The design of the enriched gardens was inspired by the conceptual model of Hebb and his followers and their work on enriched environment in which the implementation of stimulating devices in the environment had positive effects on a variety of brain functions in both animal and human studies. We applied this concept to the context of nursing homes and designed enriched gardens featuring a variety of stimulating modules. As the beneficial effect of walking outside and visiting outdoor gardens is well documented among nursing home residents, we conceptualised an enriched environment within a garden. To explore the specific effects of this enriched environment, we conducted this study in facilities that had both conventional sensory gardens and enriched gardens, to compare the effects of the two types of gardens in the same facilities. Both types of gardens offered similar interactions with nature, including an open-air walking path and an atmosphere of well-being, but only the enriched gardens comprised the specific modules designed to address dementia-related problems. The availability of the two types of gardens in the same facility is an infrequent occurrence and also a remarkable point of our study, that led us to the conclusion that enriched gardens offered specific beneficial effects compared to conventional gardens.

In our study, the better effects observed in the enriched garden group suggest that the stimulating modules are the main active component acting in combination with favourable effects provided by the garden in terms of space appropriation and mental release. Each of the twelve modules was designed to focus on specific weaknesses or disorders of residents with Alzheimer's disease. In this multimodal approach, several modules were conceptualised to stimulate cognitive abilities, walking abilities and independence. Following the 6 months intervention, we observed changes in the corresponding outcomes during the trial, which were greater for residents assigned to enriched gardens than for those assigned to conventional sensory gardens. Although we did not track the effects of each individual module, we designed the intervention with 12 different modules that individually address the specific weaknesses of residents with dementia. Seven of the modules were designed to stimulate cognitive impairment and eight to stimulate the ability to walk and independence. It is therefore plausible that the interaction with the modules in the enriched gardens had beneficial effects on the outcomes we measured, although our study cannot ascertain this point. A better demonstration could be obtained in future studies by recording in detail the interaction of residents with specific modules and examining the relationship between these interactions and the clinical effects, but this goal was far beyond the scope of this pilot study. We observed a significant improvement in cognition for the participants of the enriched garden group that exceeded our expectations.

These effects on cognitive and physical functions were statistically significant and this finding is very promising in the face of a disease for which many treatments have been shown to be ineffective. This is consistent with a body of literature showing that cognitive stimulation can have positive effects on the cognition of residents with Alzheimer's disease. This study is the first controlled study that we have identified that evaluates the effect of environmental enrichment on the main health markers of participants with Alzheimer's disease. Our results corroborate the results of laboratory studies carried out on populations of genetically modified mice carrying Alzheimer's disease. Even if the parallel between mice and men cannot be extended to infinity, the convergence of the results on the one hand, and the rather exceptional nature of the positive impact on the cognitive abilities of the participants of our study are nevertheless sufficiently interesting to encourage the extension of our work.

1.8. Limitations

Our study has several limitations. Our pilot study was not a randomised trial, and patients were assigned to groups based on the location of their rooms in relation to the gardens. This pragmatic design made it possible to compare the different groups, and it would have been technically and ethically difficult to set up a trial with a randomised allocation of residents to each group. Fortunately, we did not observe large baseline differences between the three groups, but we cannot exclude a possible selection bias. We also did not record the attendance of the participants in the gardens nor the duration of their use, and for the enriched garden group, we did not record the number of interactions that each participant had with the stimulation modules. We did not specifically measure family or professional caregiver participation in garden visits with the residents, which could have had positive effects. From our clinical experience, it was clear that although staff members at the facilities felt interested by the availability of gardens, they did not spend a lot of time in the gardens with residents due to their heavy workload. In addition, we did not measure staff attention for the residents which might have been different between groups and might also represent a potential bias. Finally, in our pilot study we did not assess the effects of enriched gardens on behavioural and psychological symptoms which are an important issue for certain residents with dementia, nor the effects on social inclusion, self-esteem or perceived well-being (Howarth, 2017).

2. Conclusions and Implications for Future Development

While some caution should always be exercised when reading study results, they present information that is important enough to be highlighted. On the one hand, and contrary to the idea regularly claimed, the conventional sensory garden, also called a "therapeutic garden," does not present any results that are significantly different from those observed in the control group. This suggests in the context of this study that despite regular garden attendance comparable to that of the enriched garden group, the participants of the conventional sensory garden or therapeutic garden group do not benefit so much in their cognitive abilities, their functional independence or the risk of falling with any favourable effects resulting from their visit to the garden. On the other hand, the enriched garden group presents significant and favourable responses on the four evaluation scales to the development of their abilities both in terms of cognition, autonomy and in the prevention of the risk of falls. Our study suggests that enriched gardens represent a new approach to therapeutic mediation for residents of nursing homes with dementia by offering stimulating psychomotor activities performed in an open-air garden setting. The results of our pilot study must be confirmed in a large-scale trial that includes a detailed monitoring of garden use by residents and caregivers, as well as monitoring the residents' behavioural symptoms and quality of life. The application of the enriched environment concept to nursing homes is a promising approach to improve the cognition, independence and daily lives of residents and to alleviate the insufficiently stimulating atmosphere of many facilities.

This study was the subject of registration and validation of its protocol with the Ethics Committee for the Protection of Persons (Committee for the Protection of Persons IDF VII, France) and was conducted according to the principles of the Declaration of Helsinki. Complementary studies have therefore been undertaken in order to extend and refine the results obtained. New requirements have been added to the protocol, in particular relating to how we monitor the interactions between the participants and the environment through the use of connected devices and sensors placed at different points in the gardens. In addition, the methodology for quantitative studies has been strengthened to ensure greater reliability of data and measurements. Specifically, we have set up an inter-site coordination committee and a method of randomization in the recruitment of participants.

This new study aims to extend the scope and verify the results of the initial pilot study and complete it with a better understanding of the relationship that the patient establishes with an enriched garden. The following questions are also being studied:

1. Are there any significant indicators revealing the appropriation of their environment by nursing home residents?
2. Does the appropriation of the environment by nursing home residents follow particular phases?
3. Are there any features that encourage or facilitate this process of appropriation?
4. Is there a significant relation between visiting an enriched garden and its appropriation?
5. Does the appropriation of an enriched garden by residents have a positive effect on their quality of life and health, in particular on their behavioural and cognitive disorders and functional independence?

This further study will have several strengths. First, the mixed method design will allow the integration of quantitative finding with qualitative assessment, thereby enhancing our understanding of the effects of enriched gardens on the nursing home residents. By involving a study management committee, this will contribute to the overall quality of research and our practical understanding and the applicability of the outcomes. Clinical studies designed to evaluate the effect of the physical environment on nursing home residents are always difficult for ethical and technical reasons. Through its multicentric approach, this protocol aims to contribute to knowledge in this field by recruiting both nursing homes residents and geriatric hospital rehabilitation patients to gain insight into the effectiveness of enriched garden interventions and to build reference points for future studies. If the implementation of the intervention is shown to be effective, the study will be made available to hospitals and nursing homes that are interested in offering environmental enrichment to their residents.

Moreover, this study will constitute a solid base of knowledge to extend the transposition of environmental enrichment principles from the field of laboratory mice to both the older adults in geriatric institutions, and to the living environment of all people.

Chapter 8

Enriched Environments: Spatial Appropriation and Health Benefits

1. Introduction

Exploring the appropriation of space by older adults is clearly a rich source of information, not only for understanding the major difficulties associated with the various forms of resignation they have to face as they age, but also for gaining a better understanding of what creates our relationship with the environment and what contributes to our identity and well-being over the course of our lives.

Exploring the appropriation of space by the older adults means, in particular, taking into account what, for many of them, constitutes a major break in the course of their life, especially when it comes to the decision to move into a nursing home.

As mentioned in the introduction, over the next few decades and by 2050, the number of people over 65 will double from 1 billion to 2 billion. Similarly, projections for the number of residents in geriatric institutions predict that this number will double by 2050 in OECD countries. This represents a major change in living conditions. In the majority of countries where these institutions exist, public health policies are based on home care, and nursing homes are generally only considered as a last option following a loss of independence that makes daily life difficult. This loss of autonomy is often associated with the diagnosis of major neurocognitive impairment (e.g., Alzheimer's disease), since in all countries over 40% or even 50% of nursing home residents are dealing with Alzheimer's or a related disease.

For these people, moving into an institution may present a dual difficulty: on the one hand, leaving their home - a home in which they may have lived for most of their lives - and, on the other, changing location at a time when they are beginning to experience difficulties with temporo-spatial orientation. Assuming that these new residents, as we sometimes hear, "don't realise the change because of their cognitive difficulties," is absolutely intolerable and disrespectful of the kind of resilience these people demonstrate. This change of living environment is often achieved in a situation of relative urgency, after having postponed the decision for a long time, and having exhausted alternative solutions for help at home, particularly that of family caregivers. While geriatric institutions have made quality of care and quality of life their essential objectives, they unfortunately do not enjoy a very favourable image. Complaints from families and residents, work difficulties for healthcare professionals, and the need to respond to medical and economic issues, do not contribute to creating a positive image for nursing homes and, consequently, to a peaceful experience for new residents, as well as to the optimal use of available environmental and human resources.

Taking these issues into account remains a major challenge for our societies, and the day when people concerned about their ageing and loss of autonomy are in a position to enthusiastically consider moving into a nursing home will mark a profound change from the current situation.

In fact, there is currently a lack of understanding or awareness of the expectations and needs of the relatives of institutionalised people. This is despite the fact that family members represent care partners who are all the more indispensable as the number of residents with Alzheimer's disease in geriatric institutions increases. Relatives thus become privileged interlocutors and partners in understanding the history, interpreting behaviours and supporting the care of residents living with this disease.

Designing, building and enriching the living environment so that a person who may be affected by spatial orientation problems can have a positive experience when they choose to leave their home and move into a nursing home is therefore an essential challenge, not only because it concerns a growing number of people, but also because it will contribute to changing the way we look at ageing.

From a factual point of view, for a resident entering a nursing home, the establishment, and in particular his or her room in the nursing home, represents his or her new home. This observation underpins the reflections and actions to encourage the development of a homelike experience (also called domiciliary approach) in institutions. Encouraged by the French National Authority for Health (Haute Autorité de Santé), this homelike experience has led to the personalization of residents' rooms, for example, by hanging family photos on the walls or installing furniture from home. This trend has also been reflected in architectural design, with a move towards smaller residential units, known as "maisonnées," where the family atmosphere prevails over the collective living dimension. Are these few adaptations enough to contribute to the feeling of being at home in nursing homes? While this aspiration to enable residents to feel at home is widely shared as a factor that enhances their quality of life, very few studies have been published assessing the reality of this feeling. Based on the notion of spatial appropriation, the feeling of being at home has been more widely studied by urban planners and sociologists as part of studies on the appropriation of public spaces by citizens.

These studies describe a gradual process that each individual goes through, facilitated by the presence of physical and sensory elements intrinsic to the space and dependent on the individual's history.

In nursing homes, the appropriation of space is probably more complex for residents affected by Alzheimer's disease and related dementias, because temporo-spatial disorientation is one of the significant clinical manifestations of this disease. In particular, we may wonder whether the process described in the literature by Fischer concerning public space is comparable for nursing home residents.

2. Being at Home - The Notion of Spatial Appropriation

The characteristics of an individual's relationship with his or her environment have been described in a number of studies. To address the notion of spatial appropriation, on an urban scale, Proshansky [189] used the expression "place identity." The notion of "place identity" is described as the dimension of the self that defines the individual's personal identity in relation to the physical environment by means of a complex set of ideas, feelings, values etc. Beyond the notion of legal appropriation of space, Ripoll [190] analysed spatial appropriation in several dimensions. The first concerns exclusive use, which leads to the placing of a fence on a plot of land, for example. Autonomous use describes a free, socially unconstrained relationship with a defined environment. Control of space describes the power and domination exercised by an authority or institution that is not necessarily the user of the space. The modalities of appropriation have been formalised in several phases: familiarization or learning, affective, symbolic or identity-based attachment (a place is associated with a social group, a use...), and the development of a sense of identity. According to Ripoll [168], appropriation reveals notions of unequal access and enjoyment motivated by power relationships.

It can be characterised by the production of signs formulated as a claim, the value of which is linked to a specific or unspecified duration.

Using a social psychology approach, Fischer [191] describes spatial appropriation as a fundamental human tendency that occurs in four successive stages:

1. Looking at a new place: a reflection of familiarity, aesthetic emotions and curiosity.
2. Exploration through physical behaviour and mobility: to appreciate the dimension of space.
3. Actions on the layout of objects present in the space, formulate a marking of the territory.
4. Nesting defines the establishment of a home.

In their book "*Older adults and the environment,*" Altman, Lawton and Wohlwill [167] describe these territorial behaviours as the need to reconcile the pursuit of individual (or collective) objectives in the same place, in order to develop one's social identity. In 2005, Peace [192] described this identity of place as a vital element in an older person's perception of his or her own identity. The loss of identity combined with the stress of the break with home was described by Pavalache-Ilie [193]: "The loss of control over the environment, the break with the old way of life, as well as changes in personal identity are just some of the changes that occur in the lives of people who move into residential communities. The intensity of the state of stress depends on many factors, such as the individual characteristics of the person (age, health, state of health, etc.), the more or less voluntary nature of the move to a nursing home, the quality of services received in terms of cleaning, security, tranquillity, etc."

For a new resident, moving into a nursing home means the simultaneous production of two processes, the disappropriation of their previous home and accepting their new home. According to Rioux [194], disappropriation cannot be formulated until the new place has been appropriated.

Rioux and Faure have established a significant relationship between spatial appropriation in nursing homes and autonomy and quality of life. However, the length of time spent in an institution was not a predictor of spatial appropriation. Pascual presented a study in 2015 concluding a significant improvement in quality of life for nursing home residents based on the feeling of control, touch technique in relation to the feeling of spatial appropriation.

3. A Qualitative Observational Study of Appropriation with Nursing Home Alzheimer's Residents

Taking into account these different areas of knowledge, but also the fact that this knowledge is incomplete, in 2022 we launched a study to assess the factors that contribute to the spatial appropriation of the collective spaces of a nursing home by residents living with Alzheimer's disease.

This study was original in two respects. On the one hand, as we have seen, very few studies have been carried out on the spatial appropriation of collective spaces by residents of nursing homes. Secondly, and even more significantly, very few qualitative studies have been carried out with people suffering from Alzheimer's disease.

The primary objective of this qualitative study was to explore the process of spatial appropriation by nursing home residents, and its secondary objective concerned the characterization of their perception of feeling at home, with particular interest in identifying the factors involved in their appropriation of the environment.

The study was carried out in a nursing home located in the *Hauts-de-France* region, on the outskirts of the city of Lille. This establishment was chosen for the study because it had recently installed an enriched garden. This configuration gave us the opportunity to assess the appropriation that residents had been able to develop with this space, which they had all seen while it was being built.

This study is a mono-centric qualitative exploratory study based on semi-directed interviews with nursing home residents.

3.1. Selection Criteria

Study participants were selected on the basis of the following eligibility criteria:

- People residing in the facility selected for the study for at least 3 months.
- Individuals able to walk or wheel independently (without human assistance) to the enriched garden.
- People able to give their consent to take part in the study and able to express themselves independently.

- People with Alzheimer's disease or related dementias with a diagnosis confirmed by the facility's coordinating physician.

The exclusion criteria were as follows:

- People not permanently resident in the facility, or resident for less than 3 months.
- People requiring systematic assistance to access the enriched garden.
- People testing positive for Covid 19 at the time of the survey.
- People refusing to take part in the study and/or unable to verbalise answers to questions.
- People who have not had a confirmed diagnosis of Alzheimer's disease or related dementias, or who have reached a severe stage of the disease.
- People participating in another study
- Any person in an end-of-life situation.

Based on these inclusion and exclusion criteria, the nursing home's nurse coordinator screened the residents present at the nursing home.

3.2. Participants

Of the 14 eligible residents, 12 agreed to take part in the study. A presentation of the study was made individually, orally and by means of an information letter, and their written consent was obtained. An appointment for an interview with each participant was made between April and May 2022. The interview took place at their convenience, either in their room or in a lounge at the facility, which was made private for the occasion, so that they were in a position to speak freely.

3.2.1. Participant Health Data
Participants' clinical characteristics were collected from the nurse and coordinating physician.

3.3. Data Collection

The interviews focused on the individual's perception of being at home in the enriched garden in relation to the feeling of well-being. One of the authors conducted the interviews in the presence of the facility's physical therapist (the observer), who was known to all the residents, so that each participant could be reassured by the presence of a familiar person. The interviews were conducted separately with each participant. They were conducted on the basis of an open-ended questionnaire that had been pre-tested with two non-participating residents, enabling us to evaluate and adjust the wording of the questions and their sequence.

Each interview lasted between 20 and 30 minutes, after a 5-10-minute introductory phase. The author gave each participant maximum freedom in terms of the length of their answers and the level of detail in which they expressed themselves. The interviews were recorded. The observer's task was to focus on non-verbal expressions, attitudes and postures, and to take note of them in parallel. When the interview clearly showed that the participant had said everything they wanted to say, and no new information came to light, it was considered to have reached saturation, and the author ended the interview.

3.4. Data Analysis

The recorded data were faithfully translated into written verbatim form. Notes taken during the interview were kept separate from the verbatim. The first phase of the analysis consisted of an analytical reading with coding of the terms and expressions used by the participants during the interview. The data were then analysed using Atlas Ti 22 software to structure the results obtained. The analysis of the information gathered was based on Giorgi's method for describing and understanding human experiences by identifying themes and associated concepts. According to Husserl [195], the aim was *"to understand the meaning of an experience, to grasp its essence for the person who has lived it, while respecting the posture of the person who has experienced a phenomenon. The aim is to understand and transcribe lived experience into explicit knowledge."*

3.5. Results

A total of 12 residents took part in the study. Their characteristics are presented in the table below. Participants had a mean age of 88.6 years (+/- 2.8) at the time of the interview. They had been diagnosed with early-stage Alzheimer's disease, with a mean Mini-Mental Status Examination (MMSE) of 20.7 (+/- 1.92). The mean interview duration was 22 minutes, with extremes of 16 and 31 minutes.

Participants expressed difficulty in qualifying or reformulating the feeling of being at home or of well-being. This is a subjective notion that generally refers them to their previous homes or to happy memories that constitute identified milestones in their lives. Four of the 12 participants had had a garden themselves in the past, and 11 of them said they liked gardens and had had positive experiences in them. For those who didn't have a garden, the experiences happened in the gardens of family or friends, or childhood gardens or public gardens.

The coding of the verbatim responses revealed 9 main concepts, the occurrences of which are shown in the figure below. The analysis of these occurrences gives priority to aesthetics, well-being, freedom and activities in the garden. It should be noted, however, that the sensation of well-being is rarely described directly, but is formulated by expressions that are its markers.

3.5.1. First Theme: The Notion of Aesthetics

The notion of aesthetics is supported and appreciated by personal criteria such as the presence and diversity of plant life, particularly flowers. Judgments about the garden's aesthetic value are sometimes based on comparisons with other gardens visited in the past, spontaneous feelings, or appreciation expressed by friends and family: "If my granddaughter comes, I'll show her. Will she like this garden? I don't know how a garden is good or bad. It's one of the first elements of appreciation and identification of the garden, beyond the fact that it's an outdoor space. This notion of the aesthetics of the space enables them to claim two feelings particularly attached to the garden: "well-being" and "pride."

The "well-being" feeling is described in different ways: either by associating it with happy memories, or by evoking the idea of staying in the garden for an unlimited period of time: "if the weather's nice, I can stay for a long time!" - or by associating it with positive sensory perceptions: "*I'm happy to be here. I like people when they come and go. The smells, the colors... .*" - but also, by expressing emotions like: "*I feel a communion with nature*!" or by inferring from other places in the establishment: "*This is the only place where I forget that I'm close to death!*"

While this sense of well-being is not described, it is characterised by attributes that suggest a disconnect with the usual benchmarks of the institutional environment. Speaking of caregivers: *"In the garden, the nurses aren't the same, they're more relaxed, they're with us like normal people. They talk to us, smile at us, listen to us; when she comes to my room, she has things to do and leaves.../... it's the only place where we think life is normal and that there's a future!."*

This return to normality seems to be a preoccupation regularly pointed out or underlying the answers given by the participants.

Did the enriched garden offer a parenthesis of normal life in the minds of the residents, in comparison with a residence described as a fatality: "I know what a garden is. A garden is life, a nursing home is death."

The notion of aesthetics, potentially a source of well-being, is also joined by a feeling of pride. This pride is not necessarily described as such, but it contrasts with the embarrassment or discomfort felt at the idea of being seen by loved ones in the nursing home room. *"At my age, I don't have many friends any more, and I don't want them to see me in my room. In the garden, you can set up as you like!"* or again: "*In the garden, I feel more at home than in my room... and I'm not ashamed of it. My son told me I was like a princess in my garden. I'm glad he's not ashamed of my nursing home. In my son's garden, I liked to see my grandchildren. I'd like them to come and see me here."* The feeling of shame is attributed by transposition to relatives, whereas it seems to be very present in the mind of this study participant.

The difficulty of appropriating life in a nursing home would therefore not only be limited by the lack of disappropriation of the person's former home described by Rioux, but also and perhaps more so by the lack of identification with the new place. Acceptance of life in an institution is motivated by medical reasons, similar to those for hospitalization; this acceptance merely reflects submission to the evolution of one's health and dependency. So, it's not a question of validating acceptance of the rules of collective life as defined by Goffman (196), but more simply of finding points of identity with the institution that facilitate appropriation rather than rejection.

3.5.2. Second Theme: Conviviality and Freedom

The participants all describe the enriched garden as a place of freedom and conviviality. While the majority of them (67%) did not have a garden before entering the institution, they feel that they are escaping unspoken rules that would constrain them more within the institution: "*... that the plants grow higher, so that I can hide a bit and feel outside this box, so that I have a bit of freedom!*" This aspiration to a form of freedom translates either into a quest for sociability, or a search for solitude. This dream of freedom is defined by the lack of constraints imposed on them either by life in a community: "*if I'm reminded that I'm not at home, that I have to do this or that,*" or by their physical capabilities: "*I'm not at home anywhere. I feel good sometimes, when I'm not in pain or forget that I can't do anything!*"

This lack of freedom is more a fantasy than an expression of real deprivation. Sometimes residents transfer the limitations that they themselves experience in their daily lives onto the nursing home itself: "*I haven't yet been given any prohibitions, I'm the one who gives them to myself.*" The garden, enriched by being different to the nursing home building, enables aspirations and even dreams to be formulated: "*It's my favorite space. I've never had a garden before, but I've always dreamed of having one. I choose the time of day to go there. I do things or I do nothing. I don't know much about planting. But it's nice.*"

The quest for solitude also goes hand in hand with the desire for freedom. The garden has passed on this heritage associated with childhood memories: a soothing isolation surrounded by plants, enabling residents to hide away for a while from what they perceive as the constraints of the community: "*My parents had a garden when I was little. I used to hide there with my sister, we had a secret corner. I could feed myself on the fruits of the garden.*"

In this way, gardens allow us to reconnect with old memories of freedom. The idea of hiding is the outline of an escape, the expression of a free departure that can be formulated at any time. This freedom is accompanied by mixed feelings, however. The desire to isolate oneself and escape an undefined constraint: "*I have to be able to hide,*" is sometimes countered by nervousness about finding oneself in difficulty: "*This garden isn't very big, but my legs are tired. I don't mind going out when the weather's nice. But if it's raining, nature tells me if I can go out, so it's like being at home.*"

The desire for conviviality here is based on the notion of free choice: "*If we go out in the garden, we're free. I don't mind chatting with Mr H... and Mrs L... they have stories to tell. We don't talk about anything. We.... we are relaxed!*" This may involve conviviality with other residents, but also with family visits: "*I like being alone, but I'd be happy if I could invite the people I love to come with me, and tell them I have a garden.*"

The enriched garden, when shared with others, is no longer really the nursing home's garden, nor is it a public garden ("in public gardens, but it's not the same..."), nor is it one's own ("*This garden, I've seen it grow, it's a bit like my baby, even if it's not at home*"). The garden thus becomes an environmental setting with which to establish a privileged relationship: "*If I can do things the way I want to. If I can invite Mrs B... I'll take part in the life of the garden. The garden has to accept it too.*" In the words of this resident, a personification of the garden is formulated, a recognition of nature's right to accept or refuse human interaction. This anthropomorphism associated with the garden is also expressed by another resident: "*I can worry about the garden! It's reassuring to be able to worry about something outside myself!*"

This conviviality takes on different forms when it summons up the memories and recollections of those who enjoyed the garden: "*Maybe my parents would have liked this garden, maybe my husband would have liked this garden, but they're dead!.*" The garden thus becomes a space of universal mediation, where people share a common feeling of liking the garden and feeling good in it.

Freedom and conviviality are linked to a third theme, that of the activities that can be carried out in a garden.

3.5.3. Third Theme: Activities in the Enriched Garden

Activities are a focal point when it comes to spending time in an institutional garden. The formulation of these activities is made in connection on the one hand with the idea and the memory that the participants have of a garden and also that of an obligation linked to gardening and maintenance: "*yes at my place I had a large garden, it was a lawn when my husband could no longer do it, it was a lawn.*" This need for gardening is formulated as a constraint requiring strength that the residents no longer have, skills that many residents do not think they have and a freedom to do that the residents are not sure they have: "*If I I have the right to do what I want there, but I don't have the strength to garden.*"

During the interviews, the investigator clarified that the responsibility for the maintenance of the garden did not lie with the residents. This precision brought relief, but did not totally rule out the relationship built between "garden" and "gardening. Some residents were still nervous about not having the physical ability or the skills to face the demands of the garden: "*It's not easy to have a garden. My husband no longer had the strength to take care of it. I don't care about it here. I don't know if it's good to do nothing.*"

However, when the participants discuss the garden they talk about a fairly wide range of activities that they practice or plan to practice. The garden is associated with the need to have autonomy in walking, but also to sit and remain seated on a bench: "It tires me to walk. If I can sit down too, there are benches in the garden. The place there is nice." Finally, residents identify that in the enriched garden there are a large number of possible activities: planting, picking flowers, making music, painting on the easel, sharing a meal, playing with others. They are intrigued by the multiplicity of possibilities: *"It is not a garden like the others. In the other gardens that I know, we walk, we look. In this garden, we can do things."*

Here we find the criteria set out by Fischer with respect to the appropriation of public space. The need to leave an imprint in space, when it is not restrained by the fear of not knowing how to do something, or by a supposed prohibition. The aspiration to leave a trace seems motivated by a double aspiration, that of the nesting process described by Fischer, but also that of verifying that the freedom to act is not constrained by the rules of the community: "*I am going to mark this garden. Maybe on the easel, or planting some peonies, I like peonies. And later we will say, these are the peonies of Mrs. R...*" This possibility of nesting is formulated with a form of bitterness when it is compared to the imprint left in her room: "*In my room when I am dead, we will do everything to erase my passage. In my room, I was not told who was there before and I don't want to know. A garden is not the same, it tells a story and it has a future.*"

The garden gives residents the opportunity to deceive the destiny that awaits each of them and do something that they feel will last beyond the temporary dimension that they identify with their stay in the establishment.

3.5.4. *The Mediators of an Enriched Garden*
Reviewing the transcripts of the interviews made it possible to identify different mediators who are part of the relationship that the residents establish with their garden. The notion of environmental mediation, described in several works of environmental psychology, characterises a transactional relationship that is established between man and the environment through a cognitive, sensory or physical component.

3.5.4.1. *First Mediator: The Memory of the Garden*
This is an intangible mediation stemming from the memories of experiences in the garden, which will open up a field of familiar knowledge for the resident. These memories are not necessarily attached to happy events: "*.../... there was sorrel, oh I don't know what was there, there were blue flowers, well there was my dear neighbour who had fun burning them eh eh eh, he was a joker that one!,*" or, "*My nephew, he went there to a preventorium in Valloire.*

Enriched Environments: Spatial Appropriation and Health Benefits

It is a beautiful garden. The nephew was cured of tuberculosis in a beautiful garden. I liked to visit."

These memories are solicited and offer a repository that goes beyond the framework of life in the nursing home to allow comparisons with reality.

3.5.4.2. Second Mediator: Gardening Skills

This skill claimed by some participants in the study, is characterised by an ability to name certain plants, to be willing to plant new ones, to remove an inappropriate weed or to have desire to water when the plants lack water. *"You have to water the flowers, I can do that. But I don't have a watering can. You have to water in the evening, I have always watered in the evening,"* or *"there have to be plants that I know, I can talk to them."*

This skill creates a complicity between the residents and the garden which facilitates the development of new interactions. However, if this skill can be a favourable factor, it is not limiting. Some residents aspire to learn and claim an ability to do so if they are not restrained by overly formal rules: *"I haven't seen many gardens. I didn't like it and I don't know anything about it. You have to have a green thumb as they say. Now I believe that I have the right to do things I will not be judged."*

3.5.4.3. Third Mediator: Weather Conditions

This physical mediator of the relationship with the garden is named by many participants as playing an essential role in their motivation to visit and stay in the garden. It is part of a close relationship with the external environment, in contrast to life in the nursing home where the air conditioning is regulated automatically. It involves making a conscious decision (or assisted by a carer) whether or not to go out, and to dress appropriately for the weather: *"I sometimes stay after dinner when it is not cold."*

3.6. Discussion

This study has shown that the experiences of the participants in the enriched garden are related to several factors including: their perception of the aesthetics of the garden, the conviviality experienced in their interactions and the activities they plan to carry out there. Each of these factors contributes to an appropriation of the environment in relation to the feelings of well-being and freedom that will be associated with it. We do not usually characterise appropriation as a concept. It is more a perception defined by certain attributes, such as pride, the possibility of leaving an imprint in the environment, the claiming of a space that feels like it outside the rules and governance of the community, and the possibility of inviting the family there and planning activities independently.

3.7. Limitations and Biases

The objective of this study was to identify and characterise the process of spatial appropriation by residents of their environment, in particular by taking the example of the enriched garden. The method used was that of semi-directed interviews. As part of this study, the transcripts of the interviews were then coded, analysed and conceptualised. The number of participants in the study and the fact that this study was only carried out on a single establishment does not make it possible to claim that the results are representative of all nursing homes. In addition, the choice of participants with Alzheimer's disease brings limitations that do not allow us to extend the conclusions to residents who are not affected by this disease. The ability of the participants to concentrate and verbalise their thoughts during the interviews, being people at an early stage of the disease, induces a limitation in the expression of their responses. It is also necessary to note a limitation in the analysis insofar as it depended on the subjective perspective of the investigator. A double analysis – manual and using information-processing software – minimises this risk, however a complementary study involving a larger number of participants and on several establishments would make it possible to explore the phenomenon of appropriation in more detail. Similarly, a quantitative measure of the frequency of visits and interactions of residents with the enriched garden would help to understand the main facilitating factors in more depth.

Conclusion

Since an enriched garden is a well-defined collective space, it offers an interesting opportunity to understand the barriers and the factors facilitating the appropriation of its physical environment by residents in nursing homes. A garden can play different roles in the minds of the residents in relation to the institutional environment and allows them to build a more personal relationship fueled by a feeling of freedom and the impression of not being so subject to the rules of the community.

This analysis invites us to identify the key factors that should be taken into account, transposed and improved to facilitate the appropriation of life in an institution, in other words the ability for the resident to feel at home. Future studies should integrate a measurement of how often the residents visit the enriched garden, along with a qualitative approach evaluating the importance of the dimensions of freedom, pride, conviviality, activities and aesthetics, as well as recruiting a greater number of participants. These additions would make it possible to usefully refine the conclusions of this first study. A future study could also usefully renew the evaluation of the resident's feelings of appropriation one or two years after the installation of an enriched garden when the vegetation has matured. We also recommend comparing this data with the residents' feeling of appropriation for a collective space inside the nursing home that has been renovated.

This next study should be implemented in the coming months. As mentioned in the previous chapter, it will be implemented in the form of a mixed study combining the quantitative evaluation of health benefits and the assessment of spatial appropriation and the feeling of being at home. We have seen that these two parameters are closely related.

All of this research and further projects that we plan to implement in the years to come will allow us to describe with greater relevance the scientific basis for designing a person's living environment so that he feels at home, and so that this place can participate in the construction of the person's identity.

It is already possible to form simple guidelines from these results in order to orient the design of living spaces that help residents to feel at home.

This work is all the more critical in that the notion of place of life is often in conflict with that of place of care:

Three key criteria essentially contribute to this objective:

- Aesthetics: This is certainly a subjective topic. Firstly, we must focus on simplicity more than appearance, which many call 'good taste'. The aesthetics of the living environment are not necessarily combined with function but more with the message and the symbolism carried by the environment. As part of our study, each resident's quest was for an environment that would allow him to escape the message implicitly inscribed on the front of the nursing home: "*this is the place where I will die far from my beloved ones!.*"
- Freedom and conviviality: certainly, the generation currently living in nursing homes presents a very different sociological profile from that which will follow it. This generation described by sociologists as

the "silent generation" is generally respectful of rules and hierarchical authority and aspires perhaps less to the feeling of freedom than will the "generation of boomers." It is up to the institutions to work with the architects to design an environment that promotes this feeling of freedom, one where the pressure of the community gives way to individual initiatives. Currently this notion of freedom is only possible, and only to a limited extent, in the space of each resident's room.

This private room then becomes a refuge or an increasingly enclosing cocoon. Residents leave their room less and less, not only because of their loss of autonomy, but also because their room becomes the only place in which their freedom is not at risk. We often forget how essential it is for everyone to have the possibility of formulating and carrying out their own projects. The physical environment should support and facilitate such initiatives.

- this introduces the equally essential third criteria, that of being able to have one's own activities. We are not referring to the variety of scheduled collective activities and entertainment which the nursing home management team strives to provide. It is a question of allowing each resident to have a space for personal activities where he can leave his mark when he wishes without having the impression of breaking the rules.

Chapter 9

Enriched Environments: Extension and Perspectives

Up to now, environmental enrichment had remained a specialised research tool, almost exclusively the domain of neurobiologists, and only on rare occasions had it made its way out of the laboratory and into the public arena.

This book and the studies that accompany it are a first attempt to take a different look at the role that the environment can play in public health and environmental policies in general. With very few exceptions, man has until now been a player who has exerted negative pressure on the environment, demanding that it bend and adapt to his practices and needs - drawing on its resources as if from a bottomless basket.

Building a relationship with the environment in which it is no longer simply assimilated to nature constitutes a major paradigm shift. Previously, society has seen nature and the environment as things for humans to dominate without worrying about the consequences, or as forces to be respected (biodiversity, climate, natural resources, pollution etc.) so as not to destroy them. Valuing the concept of an "enriched environment," if its use is to be extended beyond the specific framework of geriatric institutions, suggests a fundamental rethinking of our view of the environment. We need to escape from the "human vs. non-human" distinction, as Latour and Descola invite us to do, and integrate into urban and rural spaces an appreciation of the role that environmental enrichment can have on well-being and health. We need to break out of the pattern drawn by our social constructs, which suggest that people inflict potentially health-damaging influences on themselves in their ordinary living environment and then try to rebalance their experience by regularly or occasionally "bathing in nature," walking in forests, in the countryside, on the seashore, in their garden etc.

Our work has not validated the hypothesis that regularly visiting a classical garden has any significant influence on cognitive abilities, nor on functional independence, despite an abundance of literature based on less-than-robust study protocols attempting to assert the contrary.

Studies of major neurocognitive disorders (Alzheimer's, Parkinson's, Lewy body dementia, etc.) do not show a lower prevalence among rural populations, even taking into account the disparities in detection and diagnosis structures between urban and rural areas. "Nature," as it is offered to the general population, does not seem to constitute a sufficient means of prevention to limit the development of these age-related pathologies.

Before outlining what a revolution in the relationship between environment and health might look like, we will take a look at the prospects for adapting the concept of enriched environments to different themes and populations.

1. Enriched Environments and Older Adults: Perspectives

An interesting contribution of this research concerns the formulation of the enriched garden concept, as an experimental device for conducting scientific studies on issues of interest related to life in geriatric institutions. Publications describing the "entrenched hostility" of many families to the institutionalization of their loved ones, and the distress of caregivers in the face of changes in the health of some residents, provide additional motivation and demand to produce solid studies on ways to significantly improve the quality of life and health of nursing home residents.

The flexibility of the enriched garden concept, by adapting its enrichment mode to the clinical profile of visitors, makes it possible to build targeted responses by associating it with evaluation protocols. It would therefore be advisable to continue our research by transposing the knowledge we have acquired about enriched environments to the main geriatric syndromes and age-related chronic diseases. We should bear in mind that the work of neurobiologists in this field has been particularly prolific and has produced significant results.

The main tools for standardised assessments of geriatric patients and the relevant results of studies on environmental enrichment are summarised in the Table 5.

In addition to the areas of concern listed above, a number of disorders and pathologies have a significant prevalence and impact on the older adults:

- Behavioural disorders, generally assessed by the Neuropsychiatric Inventory (NPI), with the following indicators (Table 6)

Table 5. EE observed effects on geriatric syndromes

Standardised geriatric evaluation	Indicators Screening	EE studies and outcomes	References
Cognitive functions	Codex MMSE	EE slows down tau pathology progression and ameliorate cognition and spatial memory (p= 0.006)	McGinn; Learn Behav (2020) Menezes; Behav Brain Res (2020)
Functional independence	ADL – IADL - Barthel	EE promotes functional recovery	de Boer; Hum Mol Genet (2020) Tang; J Pharmacol Sci (2019)
Mood disorders / depression	Mini GDS and GDS	EE decreases depression-like behaviours	Sparling; Pharmacol Biochem Behav. (2020) Huang, Behav Brain Res. (2021)
Gait/balance problems - risk of falling	Timed Up and Go Unipodal stance	Gait reflexes develop better with EE rats vs control (p<0.05)	Cardenas; Int J Dev Neurosci. (2015)
Nutritional status	MNA	EE during nutritional rehabilitation enhances dendritic branching and thickness of the occipital cortex	Carughi; J Nutr. (1989)
Iatrogenic effects	List of current treatments	EE contributes to the reduction of pharmacological treatments	Alarcon; Neural Regen Res. (2023)
Pain	Doloplus	EE reduces pain perception and improves somatic and emotional functioning in neuropathic pain	Tai; Pain Pract. (2018)
Socialization	Social evaluation	Socialization combined with EE reduces stress and anxiety EE improves social behaviour	Morey-Fletcher; Eur J. Neuro Sci. (2003)

The major stress and psychological disorders observed in the older adults as a consequence of various events or practices have been studied in relation to environmental enrichment. We have summarised the main results of these intensive research activities performed on the animal model below (Table 7).

Table 6. EE observed effects on neuropsychiatric disorders

NPI indicator	EE observed effects	References
Stress - anxiety	• EE may have an inhibitory effect on adulthood anxiety-like behaviours	• Banaei-Bourounji; J Psychiatri Res (2023)
Agitation & - aggressivity	• EE mice displayed a significantly lower frequency of aggressive interactions compared to control group	• Aldhshan; Behav Brain Res. (2022)
Sleep disorders	• Exposure to EE restores sleep duration and latency • EE rats have a less fragmented sleep and a better circadian sleep-wake than control group	• Nair; Neuroscience (2022) • van Gool; Sleep (1986)
Motricity behaviour	• EE is associated with greater improvement in motor function • Motor function recovery of mice in EE group significantly compared to standard environment	• Lee; Front Mol Neurosci. (2023) • Shi; Biomed Res Int. (2023)
Apathy	EE reduces apathy and depression-like behaviours	• Meagher; PLoS One (2012)

Table 7. EE observed effects on psychiatric and traumatic disorders

Pathology or disorders	Main findings	References
Addictions • Tobacco • Alcohol • Drugs	• Environmental enrichment alters nicotine-mediated locomotor sensitization • Exposure to EE reduces alcohol self-administration in alcohol-preferring rats. • EE reduces heroin seeking in both female and male rats	• Glomez; PLoS One (2012) • Maccioni ; Physiol Behav. (2022) • Barrera ; Drug Alcohol Depend. (2021)
Post stroke	• EE combined with Fasudil promotes motor function recovery and axonal regeneration after stroke	• Zhu ; Neural Regen Res. (2021)
PTSD (Post-Traumatic Stress Disorder)	• EE reverses the behavioural impairments in a rat model of PTSD	• Sun ; Behav Brain Res. (2016)

Similarly, as we saw above, environmental enrichment has been studied intensively by neuroscience laboratories, both in terms of effects and mechanisms of action. Its mode of action is now quite well described through its influence on neurotrophic factors and neurotransmitter receptors including brain-derived neurotrophic factors (BDNF), cyclic adenosine monophosphate response element-binding protein (CREB), stroma cell-derived factor-1 (SDF-1) and its specific receptor, C-X-C motif chemokine receptor4 (CXCR4). Additionally, the effects of environmental enrichment on neurogenesis in the dentate gyrus of the hippocampal formation have been investigated in relation with the contribution of newborn neurons [130, 197].

Initial studies have validated the principle of the transposability of the enriched environment concept to geriatric institutions, through the experimental space constituted by enriched gardens. Further work is required to validate its effectiveness in all the fields of action summarised above.

To this end, the list of study programs is impressive, and will be accelerated by the various research partnerships we are developing with universities around the world. This will make it possible to multiply the number of experimentation sites, possibly producing contradictory results and making the enrichment methods more specific to the pathologies to be addressed. "Concepts are used to build theories; in fact, this is their primary vocation," as Weber put it. The fact remains, however, that the precision of a definition is not enough to validate a concept until it is subjected to the reality of empirical phenomena. Following Wittgenstein [198], Dumez [199] wrote in 2011: *"To what kinds of empirical cases does the concept apply, how far should this application go, and where should it stop? In other words, there is no concept without identifying an empirical domain of validity. Some concepts do not refer directly to an observable reality. So, we need to think about how to move from the non-observable to a class of observable phenomenon."*

In particular, future research will aim to answer the following questions:

- What is the minimum and optimum frequency of visits to an enriched garden? How many times a week and for how long? In other words, what is known as a dosage in drug interventions? Will it have a universal value whoever the patient is or will it be appropriate to adapt this frequency according to the personal criteria of each patient?
- What is the impact of interrupting regular visits for various reasons, and in particular due to unsuitable weather conditions (high or low temperatures, continuous rain, snow, etc.) when studies are conducted in an "enriched garden"?

- What is the importance of therapeutic patient education (TPE) in active participation in the enriched environment? Should it be based solely on the patient's intuitive relationship with his or her environment, or is empowerment of the patient as an actor in his or her own health a determining factor in its effectiveness?

In his chapter on TPE, Fisher takes up Piaget's questioning [200] of the role of the environment in the implementation of a TPE action: "*knowledge is constructed through action and the explanation of that action. Cognitive development results from interactions between the patient and the environment and is inseparable from action.*" This suggests the importance of building and evaluating an empowerment approach for patients in their relationship with an enriched environment.

In addition, the extension of enriched environments to geriatric institutions should address the following questions:

- Mild cognitive impairment (MCI): what are the benefits of an enriched environment for the development of these disorders? Can the enriched environment help prevent the development of major neurocognitive disorders?
- What type of enrichment is best suited to the management of depression? Is there an adaptation to be defined according to severity? Exploratory studies have been carried out on a number of modules and should be pursued by establishing partnerships with various geriatric psychiatry units.

These prospects for the deployment of the enriched environment concept cannot be limited to the specific framework of the "enriched garden." The fields of extension are multiple. They concern both collective spaces and individual rooms. The collective spaces identified and likely to be useful for the resident's well-being are the corridors, lounges and entertainment rooms, meeting spaces, restaurants and, in general, all the spaces frequented by residents, which could contribute to their feeling of being at home on the one hand, and to their well-being and health on the other. To achieve this, these spaces need to be properly designed. This includes:

- striking a balance between the resident's freedom and safety,
- not making community rules too intrusive,

- addressing the main disorders, frailties and pathologies identified among residents.

Preliminary work has been undertaken with multidisciplinary geriatric teams, architects and designers to design pilot projects for the renovation of these spaces. Longitudinal studies will be carried out to assess the benefits of these various components in the daily lives of the older adults. In the medium term, this will enable us to draw up specifications for enriching the environment.

2. Enriched Environments and Autism Spectrum Disorder

Autism Spectrum Disorders (ASD) are associated with deficits in verbal and non-verbal social skills and interactions. Individuals with ASD also exhibit repetitive and/or restricted behaviour patterns, including motor stereotypies, repetitive language use, rigid routines and fixed interests. Over 90% of children with autism show abnormalities in sensory processing, including sensory seeking behaviour, aversion to sensory stimuli, decreased responses to sensory stimuli or enhanced perceptual abilities. Some of the sensory abnormalities seen in people with ASD also occur at an early stage in the neural pathways of sensory processing and therefore raise the possibility that the main features of ASD may be in response to irregular sensory input. Autism spectrum disorder, for which several transpositions of the mouse model have already been carried out, has shown a significant response to environmental enrichment. Thus, Woo notes that after 6 months in an enriched environment, 21% of children who had initially received an autism classification based on the Autism Diagnostic Observation Schedule, improved to the point of no longer meeting the criteria for classic autism, even though they remained on the autism spectrum.

Further research will investigate whether these effects are long-lasting, and whether pursuing therapy can further improve outcomes for children who received treatment.

The main elements of enrichment used for autistic children in these studies were based on sensory stimulation, developing tactile, olfactory, musical, visual and gustatory stimuli within a playful framework. A broadening of interaction modes through enrichment is also an interesting avenue to explore for long-term action on the environment of people with autism spectrum disorders.

An enriched garden has been set up and inaugurated at the *Foyer d'accueil médicalisé Goanag* near Rennes in France and will be the subject of a study and evaluation program over the next few years (Photography 7).

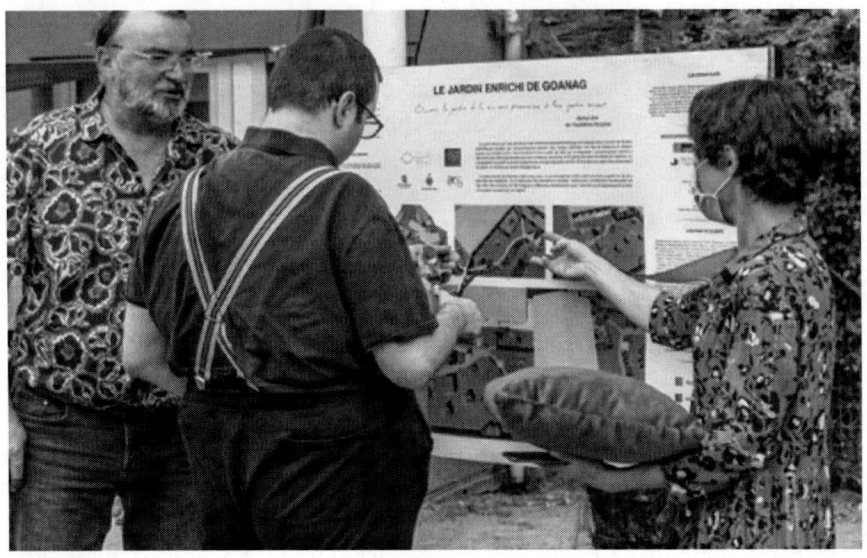

Photograph 7. Inauguration of the enriched garden in a special care unit for autistic adults near Rennes (France).

3. Further Extensions for Enriched Environments

Environmental enrichment and the research studies that have accompanied it have demonstrated the multiplicity of therapeutic fields in which it can be effective. The development of enriched environments in specialised medical-social institutions is a very encouraging prospect for many pathologies. Although our research work was originally based in geriatrics, its extensions into other fields of medicine represent a huge potential for innovation.

The following is a summary of the areas in which enriched environments have already or may in future initiate extensions (Table 8):

Over the next few years, it will be exciting to see how current and future developments in the field of enriched environments will play a significant role in hospitals and nursing homes. The question of non-medicinal therapeutic approaches has occupied the practice of medicine for several decades, without really playing a central role in practice. One main reason for this is the lack of validity of the clinical studies that have accompanied their development.

Table 8. Summary of existing enriched environment experiences with humans

	Extension fields	Existing implementation	References
Geriatrics	*See above in Geriatrics chapter*	• Nursing homes • Geriatric hospitals • Independent and assisted living facilities	*See above in Geriatrics chapter*
ASD	Children / adults / older adults	• ASD special care facilities • Schools • Home	• Sood; J Occup Therapy (2015) • Woo; Behav Neurosci (2015)
Mental and physical disabilities	Cerebral palsy Down's syndrome 21 Tetraplegic Huntington Rett syndrome	• Special facility for disabled	• Morgan; Pediatrics (2013) • Marques; Behav Brain Res (2014)
Psychiatrics	Schizophrenia Depression Epilepsy Addiction (alcohol, drug and tobacco)	• Psychiatric hospital	• McOmish; Mol Psychiatry (2008) • Koh; Epilepsy Behav. (2007) • Auvergne; Brai Res (2002) • Glomez; PLoS One (2012) • Maccioni; Physiol Behav. (2022) • Barrera; Drug Alcohol Depend. (2021
Oncology	Glioma Tumour reduction Treatment support programme	• Oncology hospital	• Watanabe; Ex Anim. (2020) • Mormino ; Front Immunol. (2021)
Chronic pain	Visceral pain Neuropathic pain Inflammatory pain Postoperative pain	*No recorded implementation*	Tai; Front Neurosci.(2021) Kimura ; Exp Neurol (2020) Yeung; Ann Surg. (2021)
Post-stroke	Ischemia – post-stroke rehabilitation	• Cardiology services • Post stroke Rehab Facility	Zhu; Neural Regen Res. (2021)

The major advantage of environmental enrichment is that it has been extensively explored for 70 years and, thanks to research protocols framed by a robust methodology, has presented significant, positive results with evidentiary value in medicine.

The next steps will constitute major challenges when it comes to associating health professionals and programme architects in order to finance, design and implement health establishments.

Such a project requires intensified research work in order to produce precise specifications and answer the major questions relating to the use of the enriched environment by patients. It will then be appropriate to mobilise academic societies, supervisory authorities and political leaders in order to coordinate such a revolution in the health environment.

4. The Enriched Environment at Home

We have explored the concepts of "enriched garden" and "enriched environment" in the context of life in nursing homes. This raises the question of adapting these concepts for use at home. For example, could we install enriched garden modules in the homes of older adults? Is this likely to contribute to the prevention of the loss of functional independence? This project aims to extend its reach to the home care of older adults anticipating a loss of autonomy, possibly associated with the appearance of mild neurocognitive disorders. A first exploratory phase of a controlled trial is being studied based on the design of an enriched mini-garden in partnership with craftsmen who contributed to the creation of the enrichment modules used in geriatric institutions. Such an extension presents two interesting questions: can the enriched garden go beyond the institutional framework in which it was designed and can it improve living conditions at home?

If this were the case, the development of the concept of an enriched environment that makes it possible to preserve the independence of older adults at home could constitute an essential transition phase to, on the one hand, improve the conditions for staying at home, but also prepare for when they choose to transition to a suitable nursing home or long-term care home.

5. Enriched Environments in City Centres

Many questions have emerged in recent decades around the need to establish a balanced relationship between the environment and health in urban spaces. These questions were expressed more acutely following the confinement of populations during the COVID-19 pandemic. The city of Tremblay in France (Ile de France region) has set up a pilot project aimed at evaluating the interest of developing plots of enriched gardens in different neighbourhoods characterised by multiple public health problems. This project aims to explore the following:

- The loss of autonomy and social ties of the older adults
- Improving food practices
- Education in the practice of oral care
- The integration of disabled children into city life
- Addictive behaviours of adolescents (drugs, alcohol, video games)
- The integration of migrant populations into supported pathways
- Detection and support of violence against women

At the end of 2019, a first experimental plot was designated by the municipal health centre of the City of Tremblay (Figure 15). However, this project could not be followed by the planned evaluation programme due to Covid-19 restrictions in 2020 and 2021. This ambitious project highlights the interest shown by cities in the search for sustainable solutions in the development of urban space. It underlines the need to preserve, in the face of these expectations, a requirement for scientific rigour, in order not to dilute the concept of an enriched garden as a a social construct.

Other equivalent projects have emerged in several cities in search of creating a virtuous relationship between the urban environment and the health of local residents. Until now, most of the dominant environmentalist visions in urban development projects had reinforced the importance of green spaces, planting of trees and the reduction of sources of pollution. Enriched environments are able to promote a salutogenic vision by proposing an urban planning strategy where it is no longer just a question of preserving the health of the inhabitants against the various forms of harm, whether chemical, aural, olfactory or visual. This involves designing a real health promotion approach around the concept of an enriched environment designed for humans. This promotion of health but also prevention of health risks must take into account the plurality of populations who travel through cities. These needs include: considering people from childhood to periods of ageing, integrating professional and student life, pregnant women, different forms of disabilities, urban dwellers and migrant populations. Exercise is complex but its role is essential if we want to promote a sustainable vision of health.

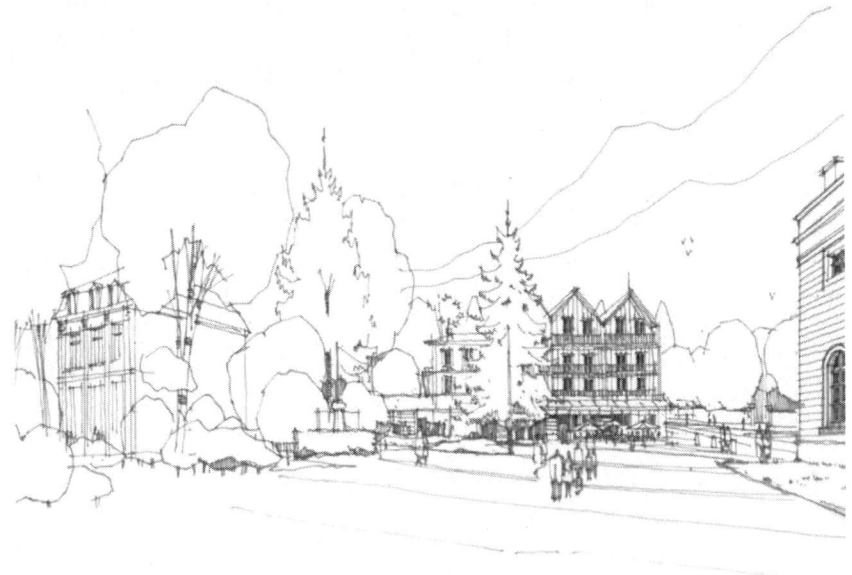

Figure 15. Environmental enrichment in city centres.

6. The Enriched Environment in a Professional Environment

The enriched environment as a means of promoting human health is a concept whose very definition is essential in the work environment. This is a notion that goes beyond the concept of the enabling environment described by Falzon [60], who questions the quality of the work environment in its capacity to support professionalization. The ability to carry out one's professional activity is used as a reading grid and an evaluation tool. The enriched environment in the professional environment is a response and an extension of questions about the quality of life at work.

The first initiatives for incorporating environmental enrichment principles in the professional setting were sent to us by healthcare professionals at hospitals and in nursing homes. We are familiar with the daily pressures facing healthcare workers. A particular goal was to respond to concerns relating to the increase in musculoskeletal disorders and psychosocial risks linked to stress.

Some pilot spaces inspired by the concept of enriched environment have been designed and developed with these different objectives in mind. The subsequent evaluations revealed a reduction in absenteeism due to occupational illnesses. Other projects subsequently took place on industrial sites, company headquarters or research centres based on the same approach: placing the health and well-being of employees at the heart of the project. One of the major developments in these projects was to have evolved from a curative approach to a preventive approach.

Conclusion

At a time when visions of the world and of people's ability to meet the challenges facing them often invite pessimism, or even what is regularly described as "eco-anxiety," it is exciting and stimulating to highlight the prospects offered by a salutogenic approach to the environment and health, based on the transposition to man of knowledge acquired about the enriched environment.

This research work is only a first exploration and forms a bridge between health and the environment. We propose a constructivist approach to reconcile our cultural heritage of gardens with a scientific approach to one of the major issues of ageing, namely health and quality of life in geriatric institutions.

At a time when public health challenges are adding up to an alarming situation, with chronic diseases accounting for 7 out of 10 of the world's major causes of death (WHO 2020) and the demographic transition highlighting the aging of the population, it's a welcome development that environmental enrichment can provide a relevant response based on solid scientific research.

At a time when the financial resources of national healthcare systems are struggling to meet the justified demands of a growing number of carers, for improved training and qualifications for healthcare professionals, and for an upgrading of hospital technical facilities, a salutogenic vision of the enriched environment describes a promising horizon for our public health policies.

When it comes to an aging population, societal expectations are even higher. In Western countries, we all know the heavy burden borne by partners, children and family carers in supporting an elderly person's loss of independence. At one time or another, we are all confronted with the need to adapt the living environment of an elderly person, whether at home, in an independent residence or in a geriatric institution. The choices involved in adapting the environment are made all the more difficult by the lack of clear recommendations as to what would make daily life easier for the elderly, enabling them to cope with the loss of independence, to continue to formulate and carry out projects, and to enjoy an environment conducive to well-being and health.

This work is an invitation to bring together, within the framework of future research, the concerns of caregivers, residents and citizens. The living environment is not an inevitability inherited from history, it is a world to be built with respect for the dignity, freedom and health of those who live there. We can mobilise a collective and humanist approach based on knowledge, proof, conviction and renewed experience.

References

[1] Mathis C. Nation and nature preservation in France and England in the nineteenth century. *Environ Hist.* 2014;20(1):9-39.

[2] Cicolella A. Santé et Environnement : la 2e révolution de Santé Publique. *Santé Publique.* 2010;22(3):343-51.

[3] World Health Organization. Top 10 causes of death from the environment [Internet]. 2019 [cité 28 oct 2023]. Available on: https://www.who.int/multimedia/details/top-10-causes-of-death-from-the-environment.

[4] Antonovsky A. Health, stress and coping. San Francisco: Jossey-Bass Inc.; 1979. 255 p.

[5] Hebb D. The organization of behavior; a neuropsychological theory. New-York: Wiley; 1949.

[6] World Health Organization. World report on ageing and Health.pdf [Internet]. Genève: WHO; 2015 p. 260. Available on: http://apps.who.int/iris/bitstream/handle/10665/186463/9789240694811_eng.pdf.

[7] OECD. Long-term care resources and utilisation: beds in residential long-term care facilities [Internet]. Available on: https://stats.oecd.org/Index.aspx?QueryId=30142#.

[8] Belmin J, Chassagne P, Friocourt P. Gériatrie (collection Pour le praticien 3ème édition). Elsevier Masson. Issy les Moulineaux; 2018. 1072 p.

[9] Möller HJ, Graeber MB. The case described by Alois Alzheimer in 1911. Historical and conceptual perspectives based on the clinical record and neurohistological sections. Eur Arch Psychiatry Clin Neurosci. 1998;248(3):111-22.

[10] Tay L, Lim WS, Chan M, Ali N, Mahanum S, Chew P, et al. New DSM-V neurocognitive disorders criteria and their impact on diagnostic classifications of mild cognitive impairment and dementia in a memory clinic setting. *Am J Geriatr Psychiatry.* 2015;23(8):768-79.

[11] Ownby RL, Crocco E, Acevedo A, John V, Loewenstein D. Depression and risk for alzheimer disease: Systematic review, meta-analysis, and meta-regression analysis. *Arch Gen Psychiatry.* 2006;63(5):530-8.

[12] Villez M, Ngatcha-Ribert L, Kenigsberg PA. Analyse et revue de la littérature française et internationale sur l'offre de répit aux aidants de personnes atteintes de la maladie d'Alzheimer ou de maladies apparentées [Internet]. Fondation Médéric Alzheimer; 2008 p. 129. Available on: https://ffpe-toulouse.org/wp-content/uploads/2017/12/RPT_analyse_offre_de_repit_aidants_alzheimer.pdf.

[13] Kok JS, Berg IJ, Scherder EJA. Special care units and traditional care in dementia:

relationship with behavior, cognition, functional status and quality of life - a review. *Dement Geriatr Cogn Disord Extra.* 2013;3(1):360-75.

[14] Gruneir A, Lapane KL, Miller SC, Mor V. Does the presence of a dementia special care unit improve nursing home quality? *J Aging Health.* 2008;20(7):837-54.

[15] Villars H, Gardette V, Sourdet S, Lavallart B, Flouzat JP, Nourhashémi F, et al. Unités spécifiques Alzheimer en EHPAD et prise en charge des troubles sévères du comportement: réflexion sur les critères de définition et missions. *Cah Année Gérontologique.* 2009;1(1):48-66.

[16] Roger S. Guide pour l'appréciation de la qualité des espaces de vie : dans les établissements pour personnes âgées [Internet]. Presses de l'EHESP. 2009. Available on: https://www.presses.ehesp.fr/produit/guide-pour-lappreciation-de-la-qualite-des-espaces-de-vie-dans-les-etablissements-pour-personnes-agees/.

[17] Reynaud F. Le taux d'encadrement dans les Ehpad. *DREES Etudes Résultats.* 2020;(68):38.

[18] Marquier R, Vroylandt T, Chenal M, Jolidon P, Laurent T, Peyrot C, et al. Des conditions de travail en EHPAD vécues comme difficiles par des personnels très engagés. *Les dossiers de la DREES;* 2016 p. 32. Report No.: N°5.

[19] Senat. Le contrôle des EHPAD [Internet]. 2022. Report No.: 771. Available on: http://www.senat.fr/rap/r21-771/r21-771_mono.html#toc267.

[20] Castanet V. Les fossoyeurs: Révélations sur le système qui maltraite nos ainés. Paris: Fayard; 2022. 400 p.

[21] Berridge V. Environment, health and history. Basingstoke: Palgrave Macmillan; 2012.

[22] Villermé L. Tableau de l'état physique et moral des ouvriers. Paris: Jules Renouard et Cie; 1840.

[23] Wilkinson P, Smith KR, Davies M, Adair H, Armstrong BG, Barrett M, et al. Public health benefits of strategies to reduce greenhouse-gas emissions: household energy. *The Lancet.* 5 déc 2009;374(9705):1917-29.

[24] United Nations. Rapport de la conférence des Nations Unies sur l'Environnement. New York: United Nations; 1973.

[25] Mittelmark MB, Bauer GF, Vaandrager L, Pelikan JM, Sagy S, Eriksson M, et al., éditeurs. *The handbook of Salutogenesis [Internet].* Cham: Springer International Publishing; 2022. Available on: https://link.springer.com/10.1007/978-3-030-79515-3.

[26] Becker CM, Glascoff MA, Felts WM. Salutogenesis 30 years later: where do we go from here? *Int Electron J Health Educ.* 2010;13:25-32.

[27] Kaplan R, Kaplan S. The experience of nature: A psychological perspective. New York: Cambridge University Press; 1989. xii, 340 p.

[28] Lewin K. Principles of topological psychology [Internet]. New York: McGraw-Hill; 1936. Available on: https://doi.org/10.1037/10019-000.

[29] Cérèse F. Repenser l'EHPAD pour qu'il devienne un habitat adapté et désirable. Les apports de l'architecture en gériatrie. *Rev Gériatrie.* 2019;44:355-60.

[30] Kahana E, Lovegreen L, Kahana B, Kahana M. Person, environment, and person-environment fit as influences on residential satisfaction of elders. *Environ Behav.* 2003;35:434-53.

[31]	Zeisel J. Improving person-centered care through effective design. *Gener J Am Soc Aging*. 2013;37(3):45-52.
[32]	Graham ME. From wandering to wayfaring: Reconsidering movement in people with dementia in long-term care. *Dement Lond Engl. août* 2017;16(6):732-49.
[33]	Fleming R, Goodenough B, Low LF, Chenoweth L, Brodaty H. The relationship between the quality of the built environment and the quality of life of people with dementia in residential care. *Dement Lond Engl*. 2016;15(4):663-80.
[34]	Hebb D. The effects of early experience on problem solving at maturity. *Am Psychol*. 1947;(2):737-45.
[35]	République Française. vie-publique.fr. Déclaration de Mme Ségolène Royal, ministre de l'écologie, du développement durable et de l'énergie, sur les grandes orientations du 3e Plan national santé environnement (2015-2019), à Paris le 12 novembre 2014. Available on: https://www.vie-publique.fr/discours/192976-declaration-de-mme-segolene-royal-ministre-de-lecologie-du-developpem.
[36]	Commission d'étude des problèmes de la vieillesse du Haut comité consultatif de la population et de la famille, *Rapport Laroque*. Paris: L'Harmattan, 1962.
[37]	Champvert P. L'évolution des structures et des systèmes de l'aide aux personnes âgées. *Rev Gériatrie*. 2021;46(6):351-3.
[38]	Havreng-Théry C, Giner-Perot J, Zawieja P, Bertin-Hugault F, Belmin J, Rothan-Tondeur M. Expectations and needs of families in nursing homes: An integrative review. *Med Care Res Rev*. 2021;78(4):311-25.
[39]	Bernonville DD. La Loi du 14 juillet 1905 sur l'assistance aux vieillards, aux infirmes et aux incurables : ses premiers résultats. *J Société Stat Paris*. 1911;tome 52:pages 216-229.
[40]	Zanetti F. Mathilde Rossigneux-Méheust, Vies d'hospice. Vieillir et mourir en institution au XIXème siècle. *Hist Médecine Santé*. 2022;(20):201-4.
[41]	Grandvoinnet P. Histoire des sanatoriums en France (1915-1945). Une architecture en quête de rendement thérapeutique [Internet] [Theses]. Université de Versailles Saint Quentin en Yvelines (UVSQ) ; Université de Genève; 2010. Available on: https://hal.archives-ouvertes.fr/tel-01935993.
[42]	Statista. Statista. [cité 6 oct 2022]. Nombre de maisons de retraite France 2021. Available on: https://fr.statista.com/statistiques/715854/nombre-etablissements-hebergement-personnes-agees-france/.
[43]	Castel R. L'insécurité sociale. *La République des Idées*. Paris: Seuil; 2003. 95 p.
[44]	Sénat. Loi n° 2002-2 du 2 janvier 2002 rénovant l'action sociale et médico-sociale. 2002-2 janv 2, 2002.
[45]	Ministère de la santé et des solidarités. Plan national "Bien vieillir" 2007 -2009 [Internet]. 2007. Available on: https://travail-emploi.gouv.fr/IMG/pdf/presentation_plan-3.pdf.
[46]	HAS. Haute Autorité de Santé. 2012. Programme Qualité de vie en Ehpad. Available on: https://www.has-sante.fr/jcms/c_2835485/fr/programme-qualite-de-vie-en-ehpad.
[47]	Marec Y. La prise en charge médicale de la vieillesse dans ses rapports avec les transformations sociales depuis la fin du XVIIIème siècle [Internet]. journées d'échanges de novembre 2013; 2013. Available on:

https://www.biusante.parisdescartes.fr/sfhm/hsm/HSMx2013x047x004/HSMx2013x047x004x0553.pdf.

[48] Sénat. La prise en charge médicale des personnes âgées en Ehpad [Internet]. Paris; 2022 p. 156. Report No.: Session ordinaire n°536. Available on: http://www.senat.fr/rap/r21-536/r21-5361.pdf.

[49] Tran A, Nguyen KH, Gray L, Comans T. A systematic literature review of efficiency measurement in nursing homes. *Int J Environ Res Public Health.* 2019;16(12):2186.

[50] Dinet-Lecomte MC. La vie des personnes âgées à l'hôpital de Blois au XVIIIe siècle. *Ann Démographie Hist.* 1986;1985(1):311-21.

[51] Hawes C, Charles DP. The Changing Structure of the Nursing Home Industry and the Impact of Ownership on Quality, Cost, and Access [Internet]. Gray BH. For-Profit Enterprise in Health Care. Washington DC: National Academies Press (US); 1986 [cité 1 août 2022]. (Healthcare Institute of Medecine (US) Committee on Implications of For-Profit Enterprise in Health Care). Available on: https://www.ncbi.nlm.nih.gov/books/NBK217907/.

[52] Fottler MD, Smith HL, James WL. Profits and patient care quality in nursing homes: are they compatible? *The Gerontologist.* 1981;21(5):532-8.

[53] Ragsdale V, McDougall GJ. The changing face of long-term care: looking at the past decade. *Issues Ment Health Nurs.* 2008;29(9):992-1001.

[54] Harrop-Stein C. Transitioning from a traditional nursing home environment to Green House homes: What are stakeholders' attitudes toward and satisfaction with the small house care environment [Internet]. Richmond: Virginia Commonwealth University; 2014. Available on: https://scholarscompass.vcu.edu/etd/3531

[55] World Health Organization. Global Health Observatory. 2022 [cité 22 nov 2022]. *Dementia-friendly initiatives.* Available on: https://www.who.int/data/gho/indicator-metadata-registry/imr-details/5206.

[56] Lawton MP. The elderly in context: Perspectives from environmental psychology and gerontology. *Environ Behav.* 1985;17(4):501-19.

[57] Netten A. The effect of design of residential homes in creating dependency among confused elderly residents: A study of elderly demented residents and their ability to find their way around homes for the elderly. *Int J Geriatr Psychiatry.* mai 1989;4(3):143-53.

[58] Marquardt G, Schmieg P. Dementia-friendly architecture. Environments that facilitate wayfinding in nursing homes. *Z Gerontol Geriatr.* 2009;42(5):402-7.

[59] Fleming R, Bennett KA. Dementia training Australia: Environmental design resources [Internet]. Australia: University of Wollogong; 2017 p. 66. Available on: https://www.enablingenvironments.com.au/uploads/5/0/4/5/50459523/dta_intro_resource1_digital.pdf.

[60] Falzon P. Pour une ergonomie constructive. Paris: Presses Universitaires de France; 2013.

[61] Loizeau V, Morvillers JM, Bertrand DP, Kilpatrick K, Rothan-Tondeur M. Defining an enabling environment for those with chronic disease: an integrative review. *BMC Nurs.* 2021;20(1):252.

[62] Nordin S, McKee K, Wallinder M, von Koch L, Wijk H, Elf M. The physical

environment, activity and interaction in residential care facilities for older people: a comparative case study. *Scand J Caring Sci.* 2017;31(4):727-38.

[63] Dementia Village Associates. Hogeweyk dementia village. 2022 [cité 12 juill 2022]. The Hogeweyk Dementia Village ~ Care concept. Available on: https://hogeweyk.dementiavillage.com/.

[64] Peoples H, Pedersen LF, Moestrup L. Creating a meaningful everyday life: Perceptions of relatives of people with dementia and healthcare professionals in the context of a Danish dementia village. *Dement Lond.* 2020;19(7):2314-31.

[65] Fazio S, Pace D, Flinner J, Kallmyer B. The fundamentals of Person-Centered Care for individuals with dementia. *The Gerontologist.* 2018;58(suppl 1):S10-9.

[66] Academic Health Science Network. Health Innovation Network South London. 2022 [cité 22 nov 2022]. What is person-centred care and why is it important? Available on: https://healthinnovationnetwork.com/system/ckeditor_assets/attachments/41/what_is_person-centred_care_and_why_is_it_important.pdf.

[67] Scott JG, Scott RG, Miller WL, Stange KC, Crabtree BF. Healing relationships and the existential philosophy of Martin Buber. *Philos Ethics Humanit Med PEHM.* 2009;4:11.

[68] Tofthagen R, Fagerstrøm LM. Rodgers' evolutionary concept analysis - a valid method for developing knowledge in nursing science: Presentation of Rodgers' evolutionary concept analysis. *Scand J Caring Sci.* 2010;24:21-31.

[69] Cissna KN, Anderson R. The 1957 Martin Buber-Carl Rogers dialogue, as dialogue. *J Humanist Psychol.* 1994;34(1):11-45.

[70] Mead N, Bower P. Patient-centredness: a conceptual framework and review of the empirical literature. *Soc Sci Med 1982.* 2000;51(7):1087-110.

[71] Lawton MP. Aging and Performance of Home Tasks. *Hum Factors J Hum Factors Ergon Soc.* Oct 1990;32(5):527-36.

[72] Moore KD, VanHaitsma K, Curyto K, Saperstein A. A pragmatic environmental psychology: A metatheoretical inquiry into the work of M. Powell Lawton. *J Environ Psychol.* 1 déc 2003;23(4):471-82.

[73] Ulrich RS, Zimring C, Zhu X, DuBose J, Seo H, Choi Y, et al. A review of the research literature on evidence-based healthcare design. *HERD Health Environ Res Des J.* 2008;1(3):61-125.

[74] Hamilton K, Watkins D. Evidence-based design for multiple building types. New Jersey: John Wiley & Sons; 2008. 288 p.

[75] Ulrich RS. Essay: Evidence-based health-care architecture. *The Lancet.* 2006;368:S38-9.

[76] Bengtsson A, Grahn P. Outdoor environments in healthcare settings: A quality evaluation tool for use in designing healthcare gardens. *Urban For Urban Green.* 2014;13(4):878-91.

[77] Golembiewski J, Zeisel J. Salutogenic Approaches to Dementia Care. In 2022. p. 513-32.

[78] Stigsdotter UK, Corazon SS, Sidenius U, Nyed PK, Larsen HB, Fjorback LO. Efficacy of nature-based therapy for individuals with stress-related illnesses: randomised controlled trial. *Br J Psychiatry.* Juill 2018;213(1):404-11.

[79] Stigsdotter UK, Palsdottir AM, Burls A, Chermaz A, Ferrini F, Grahn P. Nature-

based therapeutic interventions. In: *Forests, trees, and human health*. Dordrecht: Springer Netherlands; 2011. p. 309-42.

[80] Görtz N, Lewejohann L, Tomm M, Ambrée O, Keyvani K, Paulus W, et al. Effects of environmental enrichment on exploration, anxiety, and memory in female TgCRND8 Alzheimer mice. *Behav Brain Res*. 5 août 2008;191(1):43-8.

[81] Jankowsky JL, Melnikova T, Fadale DJ, Xu GM, Slunt HH, Gonzales V, et al. Environmental enrichment mitigates cognitive deficits in a mouse model of Alzheimer's disease. *J Neurosci*. 2005;25(21):5217-24.

[82] Narducci R, Baroncelli L, Sansevero G, Begenisic T, Prontera C, Sale A, et al. Early impoverished environment delays the maturation of cerebral cortex. *Sci Rep* [Internet]. 19 janv 2018 [cité 6 août 2020];8. Available on: https://www.ncbi.nlm.nih.gov/pmc/articles/PMC5775315/.

[83] Volkers KM, Scherder EJA. Impoverished environment, cognition, aging and dementia. *Rev Neurosci*. 2011;22(3):259-66.

[84] Resnik DB. Randomized controlled trials in environmental health research: ethical issues. *J Environ Health*. 2008;70(6):28-30.

[85] Flood D. Innovations in dementia care. *Int J Nurs Pract*. nov 1995;1(1):59-62.

[86] Cohen U, Day K. Emerging trends in environments for people with dementia. *Am J Alzheimers Care Relat Disord Res*. 1994;9(1):3-11.

[87] Bourdon E, Havreng-Théry C, Lafuente C, Belmin J. Effect of the physical environment on health and well-being of nursing homes residents: A scoping review. *J Am Med Dir Assoc*. 2022;S1525-8610(22)00428-5.

[88] Slaughter SE, Morrison-Koechl JM, Chaudhury H, Lengyel CO, Carrier N, Keller HH. The association of eating challenges with energy intake is moderated by the mealtime environment in residential care homes. *Int Psychogeriatr*. Juill 2020;32(7):863-73.

[89] Desai J, Winter A, Young KWH, Greenwood CE. Changes in type of foodservice and dining room environment preferentially benefit institutionalized seniors with low body mass indexes. *J Am Diet Assoc*. Mai 2007;107(5):808-14.

[90] Hung L, Chaudhury H, Rust T. The effect of dining room physical environmental renovations on person-centered care practice and residents' dining experiences in long-term care facilities. *J Appl Gerontol Off J South Gerontol Soc*. 2016;35(12):1279-301.

[91] Slaughter SE, Eliasziw M, Morgan D, Drummond N. Incidence and predictors of eating disability among nursing home residents with middle-stage dementia. *Clin Nutr Edinb Scotl*. Avr 2011;30(2):172-7.

[92] Bourdon E, Belmin J. Enriched gardens improve cognition and independence of nursing home residents with dementia: a pilot controlled trial. *Alzheimers Res Ther*. 2021;13:116.

[93] Dahlkvist E, Hartig T, Nilsson A, Högberg H, Skovdahl K, Engström M. Garden greenery and the health of older people in residential care facilities: a multi-level cross-sectional study. *J Adv Nurs*. Sept 2016;72(9):2065-76.

[94] Durvasula S, Mason R, Kok C, Macara M, Parmenter T, Cameron I. Outdoor areas of Australian residential aged care facilities do not facilitate appropriate sun exposure. *Aust Health Rev Publ Aust Hosp Assoc*. 2 Mars 2015;39.

References

[95] Hickman SE, Barrick AL, Williams CS, Zimmerman S, Connell BR, Preisser JS, et al. The effect of ambient bright light therapy on depressive symptoms in persons with dementia. *J Am Geriatr Soc.* Nov 2007;55(11):1817-24.

[96] Barrick AL, Sloane PD, Williams CS, Mitchell CM, Connell BR, Wood W, et al. Impact of Ambient Bright Light on Agitation in Dementia. *Int J Geriatr Psychiatry.* Oct 2010;25(10):1013-21.

[97] Riemersma-van der Lek RF, Swaab DF, Twisk J, Hol EM, Hoogendijk WJG, Van Someren EJW. Effect of bright light and melatonin on cognitive and noncognitive function in elderly residents of group care facilities: a randomized controlled trial. *JAMA.* 11 Juin 2008;299(22):2642-55.

[98] Sumaya IC, Rienzi BM, Deegan JF, Moss DE. Bright light treatment decreases depression in institutionalized older adults: a placebo-controlled crossover study. *J Gerontol A Biol Sci Med Sci.* Juin 2001;56(6):M356-360.

[99] Bae S., Abimbolz O. Ambient scent as a positive distraction in long-term care units: theory of supportive design [Internet]. 2020 [cité 11 oct 2021]. Available on: https://journals.sagepub.com/doi/abs/10.1177/1937586720929021?journalCode=hera

[100] Jao YL, Algase DL, Specht JK, Williams K. The association between characteristics of care environments and apathy in residents with dementia in long-term care facilities. *The Gerontologist.* Juin 2015;55 Suppl 1:S27-39.

[101] Garcia LJ, Hébert M, Kozak J, Sénécal I, Slaughter SE, Aminzadeh F, et al. Perceptions of family and staff on the role of the environment in long-term care homes for people with dementia. *Int Psychogeriatr.* Mai 2012;24(5):753-65.

[102] Cohen-Mansfield J. The impact of environmental factors on persons with dementia attending recreational groups. *Int J Geriatr Psychiatry.* 2020;35(2):141-6.

[103] Paolantonio P, Cavalli S, Biasutti M, Pedrazzani C, Williamon A. Art for Ages: The effects of group music making on the wellbeing of nursing home residents. *Front Psychol.* 2020;11:575161.

[104] Wijk H, Neziraj M, Nilsson Å, Ung EJ. Exploring the use of music as an intervention for older people living in nursing homes. *Nurs Older People.* 30 Nov 2021;33(6):14-20.

[105] Klages K, Zecevic A, Orange JB, Hobson S. Potential of Snoezelen room multisensory stimulation to improve balance in individuals with dementia: a feasibility randomized controlled trial. *Clin Rehabil.* Juill 2011;25(7):607-16.

[106] de Boer B, Beerens HC, Katterbach MA, Viduka M, Willemse BM, Verbeek H. The physical environment of nursing homes for people with dementia: traditional nursing homes, small-scale living facilities, and green care farms. *Healthc Basel Switz.* 2018;6(4):12.

[107] McFadden SH, Lunsman M. Continuity in the midst of change: behaviors of residents relocated from a nursing home environment to small households. *Am J Alzheimers Dis Other Demen.* Févr 2010;25(1):51-7.

[108] Palm R, Trutschel D, Sorg CGG, Dichter MN, Haastert B, Holle B. Quality of life in people with severe dementia and its association with the environment in nursing homes: an observational study. *The Gerontologist.* 16 Juill 2019;59(4):665-74.

[109] Chenoweth L, Forbes I, Fleming R, King MT, Stein-Parbury J, Luscombe G, et al.

PerCEN: a cluster randomized controlled trial of person-centered residential care and environment for people with dementia. *Int Psychogeriatr.* Juill 2014;26(7):1147-60.

[110] Simpson AHRW, Lamb S, Roberts PJ, Gardner TN, Evans JG. Does the type of flooring affect the risk of hip fracture? *Age Ageing.* Mai 2004;33(3):242-6.

[111] Chang YP, Li J, Porock D. The effect on nursing home resident outcomes of creating a household within a traditional structure. *J Am Med Dir Assoc.* Avr 2013;14(4):293-9.

[112] Low LF, Draper B, Brodaty H. The relationship between self-destructive behaviour and nursing home environment. *Aging Ment Health.* Janv 2004;8(1):29-33.

[113] Morgan-Brown M, Newton R, Ormerod M. Engaging life in two Irish nursing home units for people with dementia: quantitative comparisons before and after implementing household environments. *Aging Ment Health.* 2013;17(1):57-65.

[114] Nordin S, McKee K, Wijk H, Elf M. The association between the physical environment and the well-being of older people in residential care facilities: A multilevel analysis. *J Adv Nurs.* Déc 2017;73(12):2942-52.

[115] Innes A, Kelly F, Dincarslan O. Care home design for people with dementia: What do people with dementia and their family carers value? *Aging Ment Health.* 1 Juill 2011;15(5):548-56.

[116] de Rooij AHPM, Luijkx KG, Schaafsma J, Declercq AG, Emmerink PMJ, Schols JMGA. Quality of life of residents with dementia in traditional versus small-scale long-term care settings: a quasi-experimental study. *Int J Nurs Stud.* Août 2012;49(8):931-40.

[117] Tao Y, Lau SSY, Gou Z, Fu J, Jiang B, Chen X. Privacy and well-being in aged care facilities with a crowded living environment: case study of Hong Kong care and attention homes. *Int J Environ Res Public Health.* 1 Oct 2018;15(10):E2157.

[118] Cohen-Mansfield J. Outdoor wandering parks for persons with dementia. *J Hous Elder.* 2007;21(1-2):35-53.

[119] Hill EE, Nguyen TH, Shaha M, Wenzel JA, DeForge BR, Spellbring AM. Person-environment interactions contributing to nursing home resident falls. *Res Gerontol Nurs.* Oct 2009;2(4):287-96.

[120] Krech D, Rosenzweig MR, Bennett EL. Effects of environmental complexity and training on brain chemistry. *J Comp Physiol Psychol.* 1960;53(6):509-19.

[121] Diamond MC, Krech D, Rosenzweig MR. The effects of an enriched environment on the histology of the rat cerebral cortex. *J Comp Neurol.* 1964;123(1):111-9.

[122] Rampon C, Jiang CH, Dong H, Tang YP, Lockhart DJ, Schultz PG, et al. Effects of environmental enrichment on gene expression in the brain. *Proc Natl Acad Sci.* 2000;97(23):12880-4.

[123] Yao Z, Zhang J, Xie X. Enriched environment prevents cognitive impairment and Tau hyperphosphorylation after chronic cerebral hypoperfusion. *Curr Neurovasc Res.* 2012;9(3):176-84.

[124] Takuma K, Maeda Y, Ago Y, Ishihama T, Takemoto K, Nakagawa A, et al. An enriched environment ameliorates memory impairments in PACAP-deficient mice. *Behav Brain Res.* 2014;272:269-78.

[125] Berardi N, Braschi C, Capsoni S, Cattaneo A, Maffei L. Environmental enrichment

delays the onset of memory deficits and reduces neuropathological hallmarks in a mouse model of Alzheimer-like neurodegeneration. *J Alzheimers Dis.* 2007;11(3):359-70.

[126] Faherty CJ, Raviie Shepherd K, Herasimtschuk A, Smeyne RJ. Environmental enrichment in adulthood eliminates neuronal death in experimental Parkinsonism. *Mol Brain Res.* 2005;134(1):170-9.

[127] Mahati K, Bhagya V, Christofer T, Sneha A, Shankaranarayana Rao BS. Enriched environment ameliorates depression-induced cognitive deficits and restores abnormal hippocampal synaptic plasticity. *Neurobiol Learn Mem.* 2016;134:379-91.

[128] Downs J, Rodger J, Li C, Tan X, Hu N, Wong K, et al. Environmental enrichment intervention for Rett syndrome: An individually randomised stepped wedge trial. *Orphanet J Rare Dis.* 2018;13.

[129] Van Gool WA, Pronker HF, Mirmiran M, Uylings HBM. Effect of housing in an enriched environment on the size of the cerebral cortex in young and old rats. *Exp Neurol.* 1987;96(1):225-32.

[130] Zarif H, Nicolas S, Petit-Paitel A, Chabry J, Guyon A. How does an enriched environment impact hippocampus brain plasticity? In: *The hippocampus - plasticity and functions* [Internet]. Stuchlik A. London: IntechOpen; 2017. Available on: https://www.intechopen.com/chapters/57451.

[131] He C, Tsipis CP, LaManna JC, Xu K. Environmental enrichment induces increased cerebral capillary density and improved cognitive function in mice. *Adv Exp Med Biol.* 2017;977:175-81.

[132] Kimura LF, Mattaraia VG de M, Picolo G. Distinct environmental enrichment protocols reduce anxiety but differentially modulate pain sensitivity in rats. *Behav Brain Res.* 2019;364(17):442-6.

[133] Van Alstyne D. The environment of three-years old children. *Teachers college.* New York, NY: Columbia University; 1929. 108 pages.

[134] Gottfried AW. Home environment and early cognitive development. London: Academic Press Inc; 1986.

[135] Woo CC, Donnelly JH, Steinberg-Epstein R, Leon M. Environmental enrichment as a therapy for autism: A clinical trial replication and extension. *Behav Neurosci.* 2015;129(4):412-22.

[136] Sood D, Szymanski M, Schranz C. Enriched home environment program for preschool children with autism spectrum disorders. *J Occup Ther Sch Early Interv.* 2015;8(1):40-55.

[137] Schneider T, Turczak J, Przewłocki R. Environmental Enrichment Reverses Behavioral Alterations in Rats Prenatally Exposed to Valproic Acid: Issues for a Therapeutic Approach in Autism. *Neuropsychopharmacology.* Janv 2006;31(1):36-46.

[138] Reynolds S, Urruela M, Devine DP. Effects of Environmental Enrichment on Repetitive Behaviors in the BTBR T+tf/J Mouse Model of Autism. *Autism Res.* 2013;6(5):337-43.

[139] Woo CC, Leon M. Environmental enrichment as an effective treatment for autism: A randomized controlled trial. *Behav Neurosci.* 2013;127(4):487-97.

[140] Wood CJ, Pretty J, Griffin M. A case–control study of the health and well-being benefits of allotment gardening. *J Public Health*. Sept 2016;38(3):e336-44.

[141] Sood D, LaVesser P, Schranz C. Influence of Home Environment on Participation in Home Activities of Children with an Autism Spectrum Disorder. *Open J Occup Ther* [Internet]. 2014;2(3). Available on: https://scholarworks.wmich.edu/ojot/vol2/iss3/2.

[142] Lee LC, Harrington RA, Louie BB, Newschaffer CJ. Children with autism: quality of life and parental concerns. *J Autism Dev Disord*. Juill 2008;38(6):1147-60.

[143] Missiuna C, Pollock N. Play deprivation in children with physical disabilities: the role of the occupational therapist in preventing secondary disability. *Am J Occup Ther Off Publ Am Occup Ther Assoc*. Oct 1991;45(10):882-8.

[144] Portney L, Watkins M. Foundation of Clinical Research. Application to Practice. *Up Saddle River*. 1 Janv 2009;61-77.

[145] Then FS, Luppa M, Schroeter ML, König HH, Angermeyer MC, Riedel-Heller SG. Enriched environment at work and the incidence of dementia: Results of the Leipzig longitudinal study of the aged (LEILA 75+). *PloS One*. 2013;8(7):e70906.

[146] Rosenzweig MR, Bennett EL, Hebert M, Morimoto H. Social grouping cannot account for cerebral effects of enriched environments. *Brain Res*. 29 Sept 1978;153(3):563-76.

[147] Alarcón TA, Presti-Silva SM, Simões APT, Ribeiro FM, Pires RGW. Molecular mechanisms underlying the neuroprotection of environmental enrichment in Parkinson's disease. *Neural Regen Res*. 9 Nov 2022;18(7):1450-6.

[148] Marcel A. Le jardin du lettré. Paris: Alternatives; 2004.

[149] Mai Mai Sze. The Mustard Seed Garden Manual of Painting [Internet]. Princeton University Press. 1978 [cité 31 oct 2023]. 648 p. (Bollingen series). Available on: https://press.princeton.edu/books/paperback/9780691018195/the-mustard-seed-garden-manual-of-painting.

[150] Baridon M. Les jardins - Paysagistes-jardiniers-poètes. Paris: Robert Lafont; 1998.

[151] De Gunzbourg B. Histoire et devenir des jardins dans les établissements hospitaliers. In: *Agricultures urbaines*. Paris: Pour; 2014. p. 225-31.

[152] Huchard V. Le jardin médiéval : un musée imaginaire. Etudes littéraires Recto-verso. Paris: Presses Universitaires de France; 2002. 128 pages.

[153] Platearius M. Le Livre des simples médecines [Internet]. Paris: Société française d'histoire de la médecine; 1913. (Traduction française par le Dr Paul Dorveaux). Available on: https://gallica.bnf.fr/ark:/12148/bpt6k9722321w/f13.item.texte Image.

[154] von Bingen H. Physica [Internet]. Simon & Schuster; 1998. 256 pages. (traduction par Priscilla Throop). Available on: https://books.google.com.mx/books?id=plwoDwAAQBAJ&printsec=frontcover&source=gbs_ge_summary_r&cad=0#v=onepage&q&f=false.

[155] Jo H, Song C, Miyazaki Y. Physiological Benefits of Viewing Nature: A Systematic Review of Indoor Experiments. *Int J Environ Res Public Health*. Déc 2019;16(23):4739.

[156] Ulrich RS. View through a window may influence recovery from surgery. *Science*. 1984;224(4647):420-1.

References

[157] Marcus CC. Healing gardens: therapeutic benefits and design recommendations. New York, NY: John Wiley & Sons; 1999. 642 p.

[158] Howarth ML, Brettle A, Hardman M, Maden M. What evidence is there to support the impact of gardens on health outcomes? A systematic scoping review of the evidence [Internet]. Salford, UK: University of Salford; 2017. Available on: https://www.salford.ac.uk/research/care/research-groups/shusu.

[159] Souchon S, Nogues F, Jibidar H, Fondop E, Lezy-Mathieu AM. L'architecture peut-elle être source de maltraitance ? Un regard de gériatres. Gérontologie Société. 2006;29 / 119(4):75-84.

[160] McElvenny J. Ogden and Richards The meaning of meaning and early analytic philosophy. *Lang Sci.* 2014;41:212-21.

[161] Wilson J. Thinking with concepts [Internet]. Cambridge University Press. Cambridge; 1963. Available on: https://libgen.rocks/ads.php?md5=D33276A7E51C4A7BD236ADF4ABD79B7E.

[162] Wittgenstein L. Recherches philosophiques. Sciences humaines et sociales. Paris: Gallimard; 2014. 380 p,

[163] Gerring J. What makes a concept good? A criterial framework for understanding concept formation in the social sciences. *Polity.* 1999;31(3):357-93.

[164] Kaplan A. The conduct of inquiry: Methodology for behavioural science. New York: Routledge; 2017. 452 p.

[165] Depeyre C, Mirc N. Dynamic capabilites: problèmes de définition et d'opérationalisation du concept. *Libellio AEGIS.* 2007;3(5):2-12.

[166] Ringel NB, Finkelstein JC. Differentiating neighborhood satisfaction and neighborhood attachment among urban residents. *Basic Appl Soc Psychol.* 1991;12(2):177-93.

[167] Altman I, Lawton MP, Wohlwill JF. The environment and social behavior. Vol. 7. New-York: Springer Science & Business Media; 2013. 344 p.

[168] Ripoll F, Veschambre V. L'appropriation de l'espace : sur la dimension spatiale des inégalités sociales et des rapports de pouvoir. *Environ Aménage Société.* 2005;(195):7-15.

[169] Lapoujade D. William J. ; Empirisme et pragmatisme [Internet]. Sciences humaines et sociales. Paris: Gallimard; 2007 [cité 15 oct 2022]. (Empêcheur de Penser en rond). Available on: https://www.librairie-gallimard.com/livre/9782846711524-william-james-empirisme-et-pragmatisme-david-lapoujade/.

[170] Lechopier N. Peut-on expérimenter en santé publique?: La recherche interventionnelle en santé des populations au prisme de la philosophie pragmatiste. In: Benmarnhia, Tarik; David, Pierre-Marie; Godrie, Baptiste [Internet]. Sociétés de l'expérimentation. Quebec: Presses de l'Université du Québec; 2019. p. 219-36. Available on: https://halshs.archives-ouvertes.fr/halshs-01793206.

[171] Naishtat F. Max Weber et l'individualisme méthodologique. *Raison Présente.* 1995;116(1):99-120.

[172] Boudon R. Notes sur la notion de théorie dans les sciences sociales. *Eur J Sociol Arch Eur Sociol.* 1970;11(2):201-51.

[173] Boudon R. Essais sur la théorie générale de la rationalité. Quadrige Essais Débats. Paris: Presses Universitaires de France; 2007. 352 p.

[174] Bourdieu P. Méditations pascaliennes. Paris: Points; 2003. 416 p.
[175] Dewey J. Experience and nature. New York, NY: Dover Publications; 1958. 484 p.
[176] Grégoire F. Réflexions sur l'étude critique des philosophies intuitionnistes. Le cas de l'élan vital chez Bergson. *Rev Philos Louvain*. 1947;45(6):169-87.
[177] Latour B. La science en action - Introduction à la sociologie des sciences. La Découverte. Paris; 2005. 672 p.
[178] Descola P. L'anthropologie de la nature. *Ann Hist Sci Soc*. 2002;57(1):9-25.
[179] Descola P. L'écologie des autres : L'anthropologie et la question de la nature. In: *L'écologie des autres. Sciences en questions*. Versailles: Éditions Quæ; 2011. p. 9-83.
[180] Berque A. Ecoumène: introduction à l'étude des milieux humains. Paris: Belin; 2000. 280 p.
[181] Berque A. Environnement, paysages et milieux chez Augustin Berque. *Lab Jr Écologie*. 2018;5.
[182] Latour B. Nous n'avons jamais été modernes. Paris: La Découverte; 2006.
[183] Hartig T, Marcus CC. Essay: Healing gardens-places for nature in health care. *The Lancet*. 2006;368:S36-7.
[184] Hartig T, Mang M, Evans GW. Restorative effects of natural environment experiences. *Environ Behav*. 1991;23(1):3-26.
[185] Popper K. La quête inachevée. Sciences humaines et Essais. Paris: Calmann-Lévy; 2012.
[186] Brown RE. Alfred McCoy, Hebb, the CIA and torture. *J Hist Behav Sci*. 2007;43(2):205-13.
[187] Watkins A. Population Education. 2023 [cité 31 oct 2023]. What is Nature Deficit Disorder? *Causes and Consequences*. Available on: https://populationeducation.org/what-is-nature-deficit-disorder-causes-and-consequences/.
[188] Whear R, Coon JT, Bethel A, Abbott R, Stein K, Garside R. What is the impact of using outdoor spaces such as gardens on the physical and mental well-being of those with dementia? A Systematic review of quantitative and qualitative evidence. *J Am Med Dir Assoc*. oct 2014;15(10):697-705.
[189] Proshansky HM. The city and self-identity. Environ Behav. 1978;10(2):147-69.
[190] Ripoll F. Du « rôle de l'espace » aux théories de « l'acteur » (aller-retour) : La géographie à l'épreuve des mouvements sociaux. In: Séchet R, Veschambre V, éditeurs. Penser et faire la géographie sociale: Contribution à une épistémologie de la géographie sociale [Internet]. Rennes: Presses universitaires de Rennes; 2013 [cité 15 nov 2021]. p. 193-210. (Géographie sociale). Available on: http://books.openedition.org/pur/380.
[191] Fischer G. Psychologie sociale de l'environnement - 2e édition. Paris: Dunod; 2011. 245 p.
[192] Peace SM, Holland C, Kellaher L. Making space for identity. In: Ageing and Place. 1st éd. London: Routledge; 2004.
[193] Pavalache-Ilie M. Appropriation of space and well-being of institutionalized elderly people. *J Plus Educ*. 2015;Vol XII A:201-6.
[194] Rioux L, Evelyne F. Spatial and territorial appropriation of rooms in nursing homes. *Can J Aging*. 2000;19:223-36.

References

[195] Husserl E, Moran D. Logical investigations. London ; New York: Routledge; 2001. 1 p. (International library of philosophy).

[196] Goffman E. Stigma: Notes on the management of spoiled identity. *Touchstone.* New-York: Simon and Schuster; 1986. 164 p.

[197] Barak B, Shvarts-Serebro I, Modai S, Gilam A, Okun E, Michaelson DM, et al. Opposing actions of environmental enrichment and Alzheimer's disease on the expression of hippocampal microRNAs in mouse models. *Transl Psychiatry.* 10 sept 2013;3:e304.

[198] Weir S. Wittgenstein on rule following: A critical and comparative study of Saul Kripke, John McDowell, Peter Winch and Cora Diamond [Internet]. [London]: King's College London; 2003. Available on: https://philarchive.org/archive/WEIWOR.

[199] Dumez H. Qu'est-ce qu'un concept ? Le Libellio d'AEGIS. 2011 [cité 26 avr 2022]. Available on: https://hal.archives-ouvertes.fr/hal-00574166.

[200] Legrand L. Piaget (Jean). — Psychologie et pédagogie. La réponse du grand psychologue aux problèmes de l'enseignement. *Rev Fr Pedagogie.* 1970;11(1):44-7.

Index

A

adjusting, 33, 37, 77
adult(s), xvi, xvii, 1, 9, 10, 11, 13, 14, 16, 22, 26, 30, 31, 35, 41, 59, 72, 79, 81, 82, 86, 97, 104, 106, 112, 122, 123, 126, 140, 141, 145, 146, 147, 148, 149, 159
aesthetic(s), 13, 64, 71, 85, 126, 130, 131, 135, 137
ageing, viii, xv, xvi, 1, 2, 10, 11, 13, 15, 16, 17, 21, 25, 84, 124, 150, 151, 153, 160, 164
amplification, 94
appropriation, 14, 27, 76, 77, 82, 83, 84, 86, 90, 92, 98, 103, 107, 118, 121, 123, 125, 126, 127, 131, 134, 135, 136, 137, 163, 164
architecture, xv, xvi, 10, 13, 15, 17, 18, 19, 28, 32, 59, 60, 61, 67, 68, 69, 71, 75, 80, 82, 103, 106, 154, 155, 156, 157, 163
attractiveness, 88, 89
autism spectrum, 48, 49, 145, 161, 162

B

benefit(s), xi, xvii, 2, 4, 11, 21, 26, 28, 31, 35, 37, 38, 47, 69, 70, 72, 77, 85, 86, 109, 117, 120, 144, 145, 158, 162, 163

C

closeness, 87
concept, vii, viii, xv, xvi, 9, 10, 11, 12, 19, 20, 21, 26, 28, 30, 32, 35, 41, 42, 59, 68, 70, 72, 73, 74, 75, 76, 77, 78, 79, 81, 82, 86, 91, 102, 103, 105, 116, 118, 120, 135, 139, 140, 143, 144, 148, 149, 150, 151, 157, 163, 165

D

dementia, 3, 4, 19, 20, 21, 29, 33, 36, 37, 38, 90, 98, 109, 110, 112, 114, 115, 116, 117, 118, 120, 140, 153, 154, 155, 156, 157, 158, 159, 160, 162, 164
design, viii, 10, 13, 18, 19, 20, 25, 26, 28, 30, 31, 36, 38, 39, 49, 50, 59, 65, 69, 72, 77, 79, 80, 81, 82, 86, 87, 89, 90, 91, 99, 101, 103, 109, 110, 118, 119, 121, 124, 137, 138, 145, 148, 155, 156, 157, 159, 160, 163
designation, 60, 73, 74
dimension(s), viii, xvi, 5, 7, 12, 15, 23, 34, 35, 39, 60, 61, 66, 73, 74, 75, 78, 79, 81, 82, 83, 85, 96, 98, 103, 124, 125, 126, 134, 137, 163
disorder, 3, 48, 106, 142, 145, 162, 164

E

easy access, 87, 88
enriched environment(s), viii, xv, xvi, xvii, 10, 11, 12, 28, 41, 42, 43, 44, 45, 46, 47, 51, 52, 57, 59, 72, 74, 75, 76, 77, 78, 79, 80, 86, 88, 89, 91, 101, 105, 107, 109, 116, 118, 120, 123, 139, 140, 143, 144, 145, 146, 147, 148, 149, 150, 151, 160, 161, 162
enriched garden, xvi, 11, 12, 31, 59, 72, 74, 75, 76, 77, 78, 79, 81, 82, 86, 87, 88, 89, 91, 92, 96, 98, 99, 102, 103, 104, 109, 110, 111, 112, 114, 115, 116, 117, 118, 135, 139, 140, 143, 144, 148, 149, 150, 151, 157, 163, 165

119, 120, 121, 127, 128, 129, 131, 132, 133, 134, 135, 136, 137, 140, 143, 144, 146, 148, 149,158
extension(s), 9, 73, 76, 78, 79, 91, 119, 139, 144, 146, 147, 148, 150, 161

F

facilities, viii, 1, 4, 17, 18, 19, 28, 30, 31, 32, 36, 85, 110, 114, 118, 119, 120, 147, 151, 153, 157, 158, 159, 160
fragrance, 32, 33, 62

G

garden, xvi, 12, 14, 18, 26, 31, 39, 59, 60, 61, 62, 63, 64, 65, 66, 69, 70, 71, 72, 74, 75, 76, 77, 78, 79, 80, 81, 82, 86, 87, 88, 89, 90, 91, 92, 93, 94, 96, 98, 101, 102, 103, 104, 109, 110, 111, 112, 114, 115, 116, 118, 119, 120, 121, 130, 131, 132, 133, 134, 135, 136, 137, 139, 148, 158, 162
geriatric, viii, xv, xvi, 2, 3, 4, 7, 10, 11, 12, 13, 14, 16, 17, 20, 21, 26, 27, 28, 29, 32, 39, 52, 59, 71, 72, 77, 79, 81, 86, 89, 105, 109, 116, 121, 122, 123, 124, 139, 140, 141, 143, 144, 145, 147, 148, 151, 152
green house, 18, 35, 156

H

health benefits, 26, 67, 70, 71, 76, 77, 78, 123, 137, 154
health professionals, 17, 20, 21, 34, 81, 112, 148
human health, vii, viii, xiii, xiv, 7, 8, 10, 28, 77, 103, 104, 109, 150, 158

I

influence, vii, viii, xv, 7, 10, 30, 31, 32, 34, 37, 39, 42, 47, 49, 50, 52, 64, 67, 72, 103, 139, 143, 162

institution(s), viii, xv, xvi, 1, 2, 3, 4, 5, 7, 10, 11, 12, 13, 14, 15, 16, 17, 19, 20, 21, 26, 29, 30, 32, 36, 39, 52, 59, 68, 69, 71, 72, 76, 77, 78, 79, 81, 82, 83, 86, 109, 113, 122, 123, 124, 125, 126, 131, 137, 138, 139, 140, 143, 144, 146, 148, 151, 152,155
institutional life, 3
intervention, viii, 28, 31, 34, 38, 110, 118, 121, 159, 161

L

Lewin and Lawton, 24
light, 7, 33, 35, 37, 41, 80, 103, 129, 159

M

mediator(s), 134, 135
modularity, 77, 78
multi-sensory, 32, 35
musical instruments, 90, 99

N

noise and sound, 34
nursing home(s), xvi, xvii, 1, 4, 5, 6, 10, 11, 13, 14, 16, 17, 18, 19, 27, 28, 29, 30, 31, 32, 33, 34, 35, 36, 37, 38, 39, 59, 68, 69, 71, 77, 79, 80, 81, 82, 86, 87, 88, 90, 91, 92, 98, 99, 101, 103, 104, 105, 107, 109, 110, 112, 113, 114, 115, 116, 117, 118, 120, 121, 123, 124, 125, 126, 127, 128, 131, 132, 135, 136, 137, 138, 140, 146, 147, 148, 151, 154, 155, 156, 158, 159, 160, 164

O

operational, 76, 79
origin(s), xiv, xv, 2, 8, 14, 22, 61, 103
outdoor(s), xv, 29, 31, 59, 89, 93, 99, 109, 118, 130, 157, 158, 160, 164
ownership, 18, 77, 81, 83, 84, 85, 156

Index

P

painting, 63, 93, 96, 97, 134, 162
philosophical, 7, 11, 60, 64, 74, 101
physical, vii, viii, xv, 7, 8, 10, 12, 13, 14, 16, 17, 19, 20, 26, 27, 28, 29, 30, 31, 33, 37, 38, 39, 46, 49, 60, 68, 69, 71, 72, 77, 87, 98, 101, 102, 103, 119, 121, 125, 126, 129, 132, 133, 134, 135, 136, 138, 147, 156, 158, 159, 160, 162, 164
population, 1, 3, 16, 17, 39, 77, 78, 107, 140, 151, 155, 164
pyramid, 94, 95

R

resident(s), xvi, 1, 2, 3, 4, 5, 10, 11, 12, 13, 14, 16, 17, 18, 19, 21, 26, 27, 28, 29, 30, 31, 32, 34, 35, 36, 37, 38, 39, 71, 72, 77, 79, 80, 81, 82, 86, 87, 88, 89, 90, 91, 92, 93, 94, 96, 98, 101, 103, 104, 107, 109, 110, 111, 112, 113, 114, 115, 116, 117, 118, 119, 120, 121, 123, 124, 125, 126, 127, 128, 129, 130, 131, 132, 133, 134, 135, 136, 137, 138, 140, 144, 145, 149, 152, 156, 158, 159, 160, 163

S

scientific, vii, xi, 7, 8, 11, 26, 27, 30, 33, 34, 35, 39, 42, 52, 57, 59, 68, 69, 71, 72, 74, 76, 77, 79, 104, 105, 137, 140, 149, 151
sensory, 7, 11, 12, 19, 20, 28, 29, 31, 32, 33, 35, 36, 39, 41, 46, 47, 48, 50, 51, 70, 94, 95, 99, 109, 110, 111, 112, 114, 115, 116, 118, 120, 125, 130, 134, 145
serenity space, 92, 93
society, ix, 6, 7, 13, 101, 139
space, xvi, xvii, 3, 11, 12, 14, 16, 17, 19, 20, 21, 27, 32, 41, 60, 61, 71, 72, 74, 79, 80, 81, 82, 83, 84, 85, 87, 88, 89, 90, 91, 92, 93, 98, 102, 103, 118, 123, 125, 126, 127, 130, 132, 133, 134, 136, 137, 138, 143, 149, 164
stimulation, 12, 20, 24, 31, 32, 34, 35, 41, 46, 47, 50, 51, 87, 89, 94, 99, 119, 145, 159

T

transposition, xv, xvi, 12, 59, 72, 74, 109, 121, 131, 151

U

Ulrich, 25, 70, 71, 104, 157, 162
understanding, 9, 24, 26, 27, 41, 43, 60, 63, 64, 75, 78, 81, 82, 103, 105, 121, 123, 124, 129, 163

V

village(s), 20, 21, 35, 91, 157

W

well-being, vii, ix, xiv, xvi, 8, 11, 12, 14, 19, 26, 27, 28, 30, 34, 37, 38, 39, 77, 86, 103, 118, 120, 123, 129, 130, 131, 135, 139, 144, 151, 152, 158, 160, 162, 164